/613.0424H742A>C1/

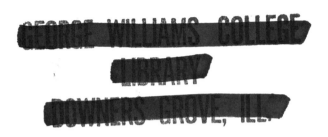

The
American Medical Association

BOOK OF
WOMANCARE

The
American Medical Association
Home Health Library

The
American Medical Association

BOOK OF
WOMANCARE

Developed by the
American Medical Association

MEDICAL ADVISORS

Charlotte H. Kerr, M.D.

A. Lois Scully, M.D.

Written by Linda Hughey Holt, M.D., and Melva Weber
Illustrations by Bobbye Cochran

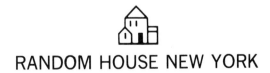

RANDOM HOUSE NEW YORK

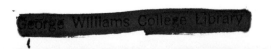

The recommendations and information discussed in this book are appropriate in
most cases. For specific information concerning your personal medical condition,
the AMA suggests that you see a physician. The names of organizations appearing
in this book are given for informational purposes only. Their inclusion implies
neither approval nor disapproval by AMA.

Library of Congress Cataloging in Publication Data
Holt, Linda Hughey.
The American Medical Association Book of womancare.
Includes index.
1. Women—Health and hygiene.   2. Gynecology—
popular works.   I. Weber, Melva.   II. American
Medical Association.   III. Title.   IV. Title: Book
of womancare.
RA778.H757   613'.0424   80-6026
ISBN 0-394-50552-2   AACR2

Manufactured in the United States of America
24689753
First Edition

MEDICAL ADVISORS

Charlotte H. Kerr, M.D., is an obstetrician/gynecologist in office-based practice in Seminole, Florida, and an Attending Physician at Lake Seminole Hospital. She is a past president of the American Medical Women's Association and a Fellow of the American College of Obstetricians and Gynecologists and the American College of Surgeons. Born in Champaign, Illinois, Dr. Kerr received her medical degree in 1948 from the University of Illinois College of Medicine in Chicago. Dr. Kerr and her husband, a urologist, have one daughter.

A. Lois Scully, M.D., is an internist in private practice in San Francisco and a member of the faculty of the University of California (San Francisco) School of Medicine. She received her undergraduate degree in Chemistry from the College of Saint Teresa in Winona, Minnesota, her Master's degree from Wayne State University and her medical degree in 1955 from the Stanford University School of Medicine. Dr. Scully is a past president of the American Medical Women's Association and a Fellow of the American College of Physicians. A native of Butte, Montana, Dr. Scully lives in the Bay area.

PREFACE

When we Americans think about our investments, our thoughts usually focus on money. Although this is natural, it is very short-sighted.

Surely the most valuable asset we have, both as individuals and as a nation, is our health. Good health is the cornerstone of almost every productive human activity. And yet all too often we squander it, either by neglecting our physical and emotional needs or by indulging in habits that are patently harmful.

In recent decades our failure to maintain our health properly has been obscured by the fanfare surrounding the introduction of a host of new "wonder drugs" and an imposing array of advanced medical technology. But these innovations, despite the many benefits they have brought us, are no longer adequate, by themselves, to meet our health needs and aspirations. Something more is required—something important.

It is now clear beyond any doubt that if we wish to continue to enjoy the attributes of good health in the years ahead, the impetus will have to come from each of us, working as individuals in our own best interests. We, as individuals, are better qualified than anyone else to act as the guardians of our health. By looking within ourselves and adopting prudent health habits and sensible lifestyles, we can prevent unnecessary illness, needless loss of vitality, and premature old age or death.

There is, moreover, a special economic urgency about all this, an urgency that affects every one of us. Inflation has pushed medical costs—and family medical bills—to unprecedented levels. Certainly one of the most effective ways the individual can combat this numbing inflation is to avoid the avoidable and prevent the preventable.

These are the reasons that have motivated the American Medical Association, in collaboration with Random House, to publish this book. It is part of a series of books called the *American Medical Association Home Health Library,* which will bring you the latest, most authoritative and most useful information on a wide range of health-care subjects. As doctors, we firmly believe that if you are given the facts, and the professional guidance necessary to understand and apply those facts, you will act wisely in your own behalf.

This book describes how your body functions and explains how you personally can play a key role in caring for it. This knowledge, in turn, will enable you to work in partnership with your doctor in maintaining your physical and mental well-being.

If you are a younger woman, a sensible regimen will not only bring you beneficial results now but also help to determine how you look, act and feel in your later years. If you are already in mid-life or older, the benefits can be equally gratifying. An intelligent, informed approach to health maintenance and to potential medical problems will contribute measurably to your continued vitality, in addition to relieving groundless fears. You will thus be able to enjoy the many new opportunities for self-realization that are opening up to women of all ages.

The practice of medicine is an art as well as a science, and it is thus susceptible to varying opinions regarding the exact procedures that should be followed in dealing with any individual patient's specific condition. Nonetheless, we are confident that the information in this book reflects the highest standards of scientific accuracy.

Let me add just one final thought: We look upon this book as an important opportunity to talk directly with you, the individual consumer of health- and medical-care services. We believe that once you are equipped with sound and balanced information, you will be able to shape a better, more fruitful life for yourself and those closest to you. That is certainly our hope.

James H. Sammons, M.D.
Executive Vice President
American Medical Association

ACKNOWLEDGMENTS

Many people have contributed their time and expertise to the preparation of this book. In addition to our medical advisors, Drs. Charlotte H. Kerr and A. Lois Scully, whose advice and suggestions have been invaluable, we wish to express our thanks to the following individuals and organizations for their aid in the preparation of the manuscript: American Cancer Society; James Beeson, M.D. (Chicago, Illinois); Sonia Buist, M.D. (Portland, Oregon); Luis Cibils, M.D. (Chicago, Illinois); Leonard Cibley, M.D. (Boston, Massachusetts); James Dingfelder, M.D. (Chapel Hill, North Carolina); Grant Gwinup, M.D. (Irvine, California); Christine Haycock, M.D. (Newark, New Jersey); Robert Heaney, M.D. (Omaha, Nebraska); Arthur Herbst, M.D. (Chicago, Illinois); John A. Holt, Ph.D. (Chicago, Illinois); Michael Hughey, M.D. (Chicago, Illinois); Leo Lutwak, M.D., Ph.D. (Akron, Ohio); Jean Mayer, Ph.D., D.Sc. (Boston, Massachusetts); Atef Moawad, M.D. (Chicago, Illinois); John Money, Ph.D. (Baltimore, Maryland); Muriel Nellis (Washington, D.C.); Lynn Persson (Chicago, Illinois); Estelle Ramey, Ph.D. (Washington, D.C.); April Rubin, M.D. (Chicago, Illinois); Emily Toth, Ph.D. (Grand Forks, North Dakota); University of Chicago Library; John Ultmann, M.D. (Chicago, Illinois); Benny Waxman, M.D. (Washington, D.C.); Gail Whitman, M.D. (Chicago, Illinois).

We are grateful to Charles A. Wimpfheimer and Klara Glowczewski of Random House for their guidance and support. We also want to express our appreciation to the following members of AMA's editorial team whose skill and dedication have been so important to the quality of this book: Linda H. Holt, M.D., Melva Weber, Bobbye Cochran, Carole A. Fina, Kathleen A. Kaye, Ralph L. Linnenburger, David LaHoda, Sophie Klim and Patricia Evilsizer of the AMA Division of Library and Archival Services. And to Marie Moore, our gratitude for the meticulous care and proficiency with which she typed the manuscript.

Charles C. Renshaw, Jr.
Editorial Director
American Medical Association
Consumer Book Program

CONTENTS

Part II   The Fertile Years

Part III Maturity: Well-Being Past Childbearing

LIST OF
ILLUSTRATIONS

INTRODUCTION

Few women in our society today follow a life pattern that has much resemblance to the one their mothers and grandmothers knew. Indeed, many women find their life—and their attitudes toward it—astonishingly different from what, in girlhood, they planned or anticipated for themselves.

This was not the case in past generations. Except in times of historic upheavals, such as those involving war or pestilence, a woman could more or less rely on walking in the paths of her predecessors.

Those paths have now largely been obliterated, and we can no longer either live or think in the same way as women of even very recent generations. Among the ideas that have profoundly changed are those regarding a woman's body and the way it is dealt with in terms of medical and health practice.

The key to all this change? Modern contraception, which more than any other single factor has made the liberation of women not only possible, but inevitable. "Anatomy is destiny," said Freud, no doubt referring to women in particular. True, but today anatomy no longer quite so severely limits our destiny.

The fact that today millions of women have a measure of control over the consequences of sexual activity has amounted to a veritable biological revolution, touching almost every life, changing the entire course of society. There is no avoiding the widespread effects of this biological revolution, no escape from the new responsibilities, no turning back to yesterday's no-choice position. Even if a woman chooses to be a homemaker and mother like her own mother and grandmother before her, there's one critical difference: she *chooses*. For her mother and grandmother, there was seldom any alternative. Now that we women have options, we have a greater than ever responsibility to exercise those choices fully and wisely. A primary area of that responsibility is health.

In the following chapters we will explore women's health-care options, using the experience of women physicians who, working with the AMA, have had the primary responsibility for the content of this book. All of us are actively engaged in health care and are at the same time consumers of health care, sharing with you, the woman reader, the possession of a female body and the phases of a woman's physical life.

This will be a "reason why" book as well as a "how to" book. The changing roles for women in our society have brought important changes in the way women regard their bodies and their minds, and inevitably, in the ways they take care of their health and deal with physical problems. Also in this book, some outworn medical attitudes toward women will be examined—mainly for the purpose of discarding them.

We hope this book will bring you, the reader:

- Increased knowledge of your body and the way it functions
- More skill in self-care: knowing which symptoms or problems you can take care of yourself; learning how to prevent health problems; and being able to tell when you need professional medical help
- A better understanding of professional medical care and of ways to work effectively with your physician in the prevention and management of illness

We hope you will be able to use the book in two ways: First, read it through for a full view of the concept of the well woman, the way she is constructed, the way she functions and how she can best care for her body; and second, go back to it from time to time, for reference to specific points and topics.

In addition, we hope this book will be fun and thought-provoking; we hope that it will bring moments of wonder at what women have experienced (and survived) in the past; and we also hope it will lead you to share our confidence in ever-improving chances for health and well-being, now and tomorrow.

Some years ago, hospitals started using the term "well-baby clinic" to identify the department to which you took your child for regular checkups, inoculations and health advice. The name has a lift to it; it means medical attention for those currently in good health—the kind of attention that is vitally necessary if being well is to be an ongoing condition.

We think "well woman" expresses the purpose of this book. To continue enjoying the blessing of health, a woman at any age needs to know a great deal about her body and the ways it functions. She needs to know what to do to stay well, what minor ailments she can manage by herself, which symptoms ought to be taken up with her physician. She especially needs to know how to avoid health problems, for preventive care today is to a great extent in one's own hands. This book, then, is about living well, in the literal sense.

We will consider and discuss the "well woman" as a whole person, but will place major emphasis on her essentially female aspects: the reproductive system, the female life cycles and the health issues that affect women in particular.

Linda Hughey Holt, M.D.
Charlotte H. Kerr, M.D.
A. Lois Scully, M.D.

PART I

THROUGHOUT YOUR LIFE

Part I of this book is, in a sense, a map. We will explore and describe the boundaries of the female body, some of its organic territories, and many major points of interest.

We include not only the body's geography but some of its natural history as well, for here we consider health matters that may affect a woman at any time in her adult life. In Parts II and III we will take up specific life cycles, such as the beginning of fertility, the fertile years, and the mature years past childbearing; here, we first consider the health factors that touch all of us at all ages.

"What your body is at fifteen, God gave you; at fifty, what you made of it," a wise person once said. In Chapter 1 we will look at the structure of the female body, the ways it functions and the ways in which it differs from the male body. Next we will discuss the ground rules for lifelong health, including the way you eat, work, sleep and exercise. These habits have direct and lasting effects on your health and well-being. In the third chapter we will discuss how to make the most of medical services, how to choose a private physician and work with him to keep yourself in the best of health. Finally we will discuss the most common symptoms and what they may be trying to tell you, and offer advice on which problems you can manage yourself and which ones need medical attention.

1

THE FEMALE BODY

. . . a rag and a bone and a hank of hair . . .
And a woman is only a woman, but a good cigar is
a smoke.

Endlessly quoted for almost a century now, Rudyard Kipling's barracks-room characterizations of woman wouldn't identify her very clearly for any visitor from outer space—especially one who is somewhat of a physiologist and wants some basic physical facts. But the following generalities might help:

She has more than 200 distinct bones, about two and one half yards of skin, more than 600 separate muscles made up of a quarter-billion fibers, and she contains four to five quarts of blood. At the periphery of her blood's circulation there are so many fine, hairlike capillary vessels that if they were joined, they could be wound several times around the earth. Equally minute are the 300 million air sacs in her lungs. Her stomach, with its capacity of four to five pints, contains about 35 million glands that dispense juices necessary to break down and liquefy the food from which she subsequently extracts energy.

Those are merely a few points to illustrate the complexity and wonder of the human body. In addition it is animated by electrical charges, as in the brain, heart and nerves. It is built of cells so intricate and specialized that a cell biologist can find a universe to explore in any single one; and it manufactures and uses a range of hormones, enzymes and other substances so subtly interrelated that we have only begun to unwind their chemistry and functions.

The male and female human anatomies differ in a number of ways. The woman is generally shorter than the male and generally lighter in frame and weight. The male physique typically has greater muscular strength. The female's pelvic bones are broader and more flared in shape, more widely spaced and carried at a different angle, designed to accommodate pregnancy and birth. Female breasts tend to be prominent and well developed; the corresponding structure in the male is fairly flat and rudimentary. The female body appears more curved and rounded than that of the male because her muscles are more likely to be sheathed in a layer of fatty tissue just beneath the skin. Finally, the most pronounced differences of all are those of the male and female reproductive systems; his for generating sperm and impregnation, hers for egg producing, nourishing and bearing.

A researcher in gender identity, John Money, Ph.D., of Johns Hopkins University in Baltimore, reminds us that sex differences between males and females are not absolute, but arrayed along a continuum. For example, there are no totally "male" or "female" hormones; sex hormones are present in everyone, but the predominance of androgen or estrogen can define male or female functioning. Even the chromosomes are not absolute determinants of gender, Dr. Money points out, since the XX (female) and XY (male) patterns are subject to variants such as XXX, XXY, XXXY, XXYY, XYY, X, and other combinations or mosaics. And as he has emphasized in many books and articles, our sexual identity is also determined by our culture and society. So it's not surprising that secondary sexual characteristics, such as facial and body hair, pitch of the voice, muscularity and stature occur along a very wide range for both sexes. The female body we discuss and illustrate in the following pages is the most typical and representative.

To begin getting acquainted with the physical being we intend to study and learn about in this book, let us take a brief tour of some of the body's major systems, remembering that the various tissues and organs don't have lines dividing them. For example, the mouth, esophagus, stomach and gut are essentially one piece with different processes going on at different points. Though we look at our anatomical "systems" as separate parts, we know they really are quite inseparable and that we function largely as a whole organism.

This is an important concept when we consider the maintenance of our health; the body generally cannot be "fixed" in the same way we tinker with an errant carburetor or spark plug in an automobile. We need to take care of the entire body—as a whole.

Bones

Many of us tend to think of the skeleton as an inert supporting framework, and of bones as something hard and semipermanent. Not so. The cells of our bony tissues are in constant flux, breaking down and being rebuilt. The skeleton, in fact, is completely renewed about every two years.

Bone is light (only one fifth of the body's weight) and strong. Not only does it serve as the frame that makes movement possible (without a skeleton we would be a soft heap of flesh) and as a shelter for fragile organs such as the brain, lungs and intestines; it is also a storehouse for minerals needed throughout the body, and its marrow has the ability to make red blood cells. About half the bone material is mineral, chiefly calcium. The rest is water and collagen, a remarkable protein substance present not only in bone but in almost every body tissue including skin, connective parts and the crystal-clear outer window of the eye.

Keeping your bones in good health requires an adequate diet—and adequate physical activity as well. Without exercise and weight-bearing stress, the bones can lose their minerals, soften and break. When a limb is put into a cast so that a fracture can heal, it may lose as much as half its calcium during the immobile period. This loss, however, is replenished rapidly once regular activity is resumed.

How does exercise strengthen hard, rigid bone? Grant Gwinup, M.D., professor of medicine and endocrinology at the University of California at Irvine, explains it: "Stress on a bone actually bends it slightly, setting up electrical currents that lead to deposition of new material. Activity literally sends a charge through your bones, an electrochemical action that keeps the bone rebuilding itself."

Among the dietary elements that support bone health is calcium. It is important to have not only enough calcium but a balance of calcium to phosphorus. Other dietary ingredients essential to bone health include vitamin D (it activates calcium metabolism), adequate protein and a minute amount of fluoride. Pregnant and nursing women need a good deal extra protein and calcium to maintain the maternal skeleton (which, if necessary, will deplete its own calcium stores to supply the growing fetus) and to provide building materials for the infant skeleton. See Chapter 6 for more about this.

Another time during a woman's life when she should pay special attention to bone health is during the climacteric (menopause), when there is the potential threat of osteoporosis, or thinning and weakened bones. (This will be discussed in Chapter 13.) It should be noted here, however, that older women need more calcium, not, as is commonly believed, less of it than in their earlier years.

Muscles

Those 600-plus muscles we mentioned make up about 40 percent of your body's weight. Muscles are of three major kinds: the smooth *involuntary* muscles that work without your conscious direction, operating blood vessels, producing intestinal motion, giving motion to other organs, even down to the tiny drawstring that dilates or contracts the iris of your eye; the *heart muscle,* a type by itself— involuntary also, but made of interlocked fibers knitted together for squeeze-and-release action; and the *skeletal,* or *striated,* muscles, so named because they appear gaily striped beneath the microscope, their light and dark bands ceaselessly flexing. This last group is comprised of *voluntary* muscles; we can direct them as we choose, and we can exercise and develop them for strength, suppleness and endurance.

Now a physiological surprise: Moving the body is not the only function of the skeletal muscles. They are also a great metabolic organ, storing protein and regulating the levels of proteins and sugars in the bloodstream. The liver, weighing barely three pounds, cannot possibly do all that is needed to break down proteins, build them anew, convert amino acids into glucose and keep nutrients balanced in the blood. The muscle mass, according to Peter Maxwell Daniel and fellow colleagues of the Royal College of Surgeons in London, achieves two to three times as much protein turnover as does the liver. The London researchers believe that the metabolic process of skeletal muscles is as vital as their other, more obvious functions: providing motion and power, and keeping the body erect.

Muscles make action possible, but they urgently need action in order to maintain what we know as muscle tone. The constant, almost imperceptible motion of the striated muscle fibers may be the source of the name *musculus* ("little mouse") for the rippling, running action of muscle beneath the skin.

Today women are no longer concerned that physical activity will cause bunchy, brawny muscles. For one thing, the sweeping popularity of sports and exercise has vividly demonstrated that active women look very good indeed. Endocrinologists explain that whereas in the male body the hormone testosterone contributes to knotty, bulging muscles, the female body, with much smaller amounts of testosterone and larger amounts of female hormones, develops smooth curves.

Lungs

Millions upon millions of alveoli (the air sacs of the lungs made of incredibly delicate, one-cell-thick tissue) work unceasingly throughout life, moving oxygen into the bloodstream, removing carbon dioxide and other wastes, constantly cleaning and sweeping out. The insides of your lungs have a working area that adds up to about 27 by 30 feet. The allowance of air sacs is so generous that many people live very comfortably after surgical removal of a great deal of lung tissue, even of an entire lung. Air pollutants, including cigarette smoke, and various lung diseases can impair lung function substantially before life actually is threatened. Still, we generally feel best when our lungs are working in a normal, healthy manner.

Should we "do" anything, such as take up breathing exercises, to benefit the lungs? There's no need for it, according to pulmonary authorities. Normal breathing is automatic, and the lungs themselves have no muscles to contract. Exercise is very good for the body as a whole; it can build up the chest muscles, strengthen skeletal muscles, and tune up the heart and blood vessels. But conditioning does very little to expand the lungs.

Sonia Buist, M.D., of the University of Oregon Health Sciences Center, Department of Physiology, explains how breathing is controlled. Mechanical receptors in the chest wall, muscles and diaphragm report to the brain centers on the degree of inflation of the lungs. Also, chemical receptors in certain blood vessels and in the brain report the amounts of waste products, principally carbon dioxide, in the blood. "If you hold your breath, the carbon dioxide will increase," says Dr. Buist. "Immediately the chemical receptors sense it, and immediately they send a message to the brain saying 'For heaven's sake, take a breath.' Then, when you take the breath, the receptors get stretched, so they send a message saying 'You've breathed in enough; breathe out now.' The process is quite complex, but at the same time it's automatic. And the chemical balance is maintained very, very closely. It's just body wisdom, and we don't have to think it out at all."

Of course, human beings are able to control breathing deliberately, even if it isn't necessary. What about those "deep breathing exercises"? "They won't do much more than hyperventilate you, which makes you feel dizzy or faint," says Dr. Buist. If you carry hyperventilation to an extreme, you will probably lose consciousness. Thereupon your automatic breathing control will take over and correct the situation.

Health authorities are virtually in total agreement that cigarette smoking is a menace to pulmonary health, in that it is a high risk factor in lung cancer and heart disease as well as a host of other conditions, including the dreaded emphysema, in which exhaling becomes difficult. Chronic obstructive lung diseases, such as emphysema and chronic bronchitis, strike smokers far more often than nonsmokers. Special exercises are often recommended for emphysema sufferers—not to strengthen lung tissue, but to improve total body health in the hope of slowing the progress of the disease.

Another problem receiving increased attention is air pollution. Almost all fitness experts now recommend that joggers stay inside during pollution alerts; the potential damage can easily outweigh the benefits.

Breasts

"Hemispherical eminences"—as described in the classic text *Gray's Anatomy*—the female breasts are made up of milk glands, fibrous connective tissue, fatty tissue and blood vessels (see illustration).

BREAST GLANDULAR STRUCTURE

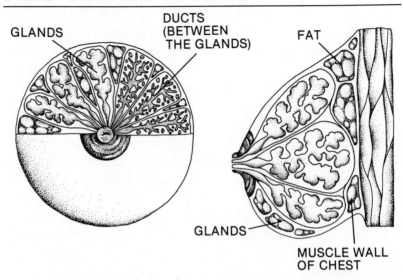

GLANDS

DUCTS
(BETWEEN
THE GLANDS)

FAT

GLANDS

MUSCLE WALL
OF CHEST

Complex of glands, ducts and fatty tissue which comprise the breast.

The milk-producing glands, shaped like many clusters of tiny grapes, are connected into a duct system, small tubes leading into larger ones, and finally into a series of canals proceeding toward the center and enlarging into ampules, bottle-shaped swellings that serve as milk reservoirs. These lie just beneath the areola, the pink-brown disk of skin at the nipple base. In lactation, milk is drawn from the reservoirs through many small openings in the tip of the nipple.

The only muscles within the breast are tiny ones that cause the nipple to grow erect. The shape of the breasts is primarily maintained by fibers called Cooper's ligaments, leading from the front of the breast back to the chest wall.

Breasts enlarge greatly during pregnancy, as milk glands develop. For many women, breasts also enlarge or become engorged during the middle of the menstrual cycle. Breasts are responsive to the body's hormones, to the presence of one's baby, and to sexual excitement.

Breast cancer is diagnosed in about 100,000 women each year. Because breast cancer is highly curable if detected and treated early, it is of utmost importance to examine one's own breasts regularly and to have them examined by the doctor at every office visit. (See Chapter 14 for more information about breast cancer and self-examination of breasts.)

Nervous System

To many, the most awe-inspiring structure in all nature is the human nervous system. It consists of the brain, the spinal cord and myriad branches of nerves radiating to the outer surfaces of the body. This system, which allows us to think, move, touch and experience life in its entirety, also commands every body process, largely without the conscious control we know as "thinking."

Atop the nervous system sits the brain. It weighs three pounds, more or less, and includes the thinking apparatus itself, called the cerebrum. Beneath the cerebrum are several other brain segments, which house the ancient control lines—some say the primordial memories—that govern bodily functions and consciousness itself. Beneath these brain segments there are about 18 inches of spinal cord, made of gray and white tissue like that in the brain and lying almost loosely in its flexible carved tunnel of bone. Branching out from the spinal cord are nerves that carry their messages throughout the body—registering sights and smells, motion, pain and pleasure. Electrical charges hum through these lines to regulate blood flow, to squeeze and stretch muscle fibers, to keep the rhythm of processes like digestion. Nerve cells, called neurons, are the basic units of these lines; it is estimated that every one of us has ten billion of them.

One of the latest surprises in scientific research is the discovery of the brain's drug-manufacturing capability. In the early 1970s, scientists began to identify sites on brain cells acting as "receptors" for chemical substances that stimulate various kinds of brain activity. When receptors were found that fitted the morphine molecule, scientists saw a clue: the human brain could not have evolved a receiving device for a man-made substance; therefore, a chemical made by the body itself must exist. And it had to be an opiate-like chemical that would modify pain impulses. They found the chemical, and the family of brain-made chemical relatives called enkephalins and endorphins were discovered.

Evidence is building up showing that nutrition can influence brain function and that folklore about "brain foods" may indeed bear some relation to scientific fact. As researchers explain it, the brain cells' ability to make and release several chemicals depends directly on the concentration of amino acids and choline (one of the B-complex vitamins) in the blood—and therefore on the composition of the latest meal. Among food substances now being explored for their effects on memory and other thinking processes, as well as on sleep and pain control, are amino acids such as tryptophan and tyrosine, as well as choline and lecithin (they are found in milk and other protein foods). During the present decade we may witness—and take part in—exciting advances in nutrition for improved mental function.

Circulatory System

In ancient days the heart was believed to be the dwelling place of the soul and the passions; even today we continue to use expressions reflecting that belief. We know things "deep in our hearts"; we learn "by heart" those items we commit to memory; our loved ones are "dear to my heart." The heart may not be the storage place for fond memories and feelings, but it is no less remarkable as a muscular pump, and the blood vessels that make up the vascular system perform near-miracles in fluid engineering. The blood itself—that river of life associated with nearly as much folklore as the heart—carries out countless chores while moving through the miles of large and small blood vessels in our bodies. For some reason, the annals of legend, poetry and song have seldom celebrated the veins and arteries of heroes and heroines—only their throbbing hearts.

Heart disease is responsible for a million deaths in the United States each year, making it our leading killer disease. But the death rate is on a downward trend and has been for some years. Possible reasons for this brightening picture include better emergency hospital care for heart-attack victims, saving lives that earlier might have been lost; more and better heart-surgery techniques; and improved management of high blood pressure, with more cases detected and treated. Also, there is now more public awareness of preventive health measures such as quitting cigarettes and getting adequate exercise.

Women have a lower risk of heart attacks than men. It is believed that the estrogen in women's bodies may act as a protector against coronary disease. After menopause, when the estrogen supply drops off, the woman's heart-disease risk increases to nearly that of her male counterpart.

Some health leaders speculate that since an increasing number of women are in high-pressure jobs, smoke cigarettes and use "the pill," there will soon be a near-equality of heart-disease risk in both sexes. But at least one report based on data from the immense Framingham Study (which involves an entire Massachusetts community) shows that women working full-time outside the home are at no greater risk of contracting coronary heart disease than women who remain at home. The report finds, however, that women performing certain boring tasks such as clerical work, those with extra family responsibilities in addition to jobs, and those in dead-end, frustrating occupations were more likely to get heart disease. As might be expected, it's not the fact of being employed but being under unrelieved stress that hurts.

High blood pressure, obesity, smoking and lack of exercise are risk factors for heart disease that you can control. Others (you may not be able to change them, but you can reduce them by instituting good health habits and being alert to signals) include aging, heredity, ethnic or racial origin and your early environment.

All women should have blood-pressure readings regularly and should be on the alert for any changes or trends that develop. Black women need to be especially watchful, since the incidence of hypertension—high blood pressure—is considerably greater both in black men and women than in whites.

It is a misconception that your blood pressure is supposed to rise as you grow older, says the National High Blood Pressure Education Program. In fact, your blood pressure should not exceed 140/90 at any age. If it does, you should take steps to lower it by restricting the use of salt, by reducing if you weigh too much, and by consulting your doctor about any need for medication. In almost all cases the above steps, in addition to possibly using a mild diuretic, will bring down the blood pressure to a satisfactory level. (The following chapter contains more information about nutrition, exercise, blood-iron levels and other factors that can help you maintain a healthy circulatory system.)

Digestive System

We are generally aware of our digestive apparatus only when it's misbehaving. All we ask of our stomach and intestines is quiet, pain-free functioning without any signs of disorder, along with a perfectly poised metabolism so we neither gain nor lose weight. We would greatly prefer not having intestinal cramps and diarrhea when we're going through an emotional crisis or some stress-producing event, but as you probably know, our insides are merely sympathetic and trying to help, even though the effort seems misplaced.

When you get angry, your stomach lining gets angry too; it flushes dark-red and pours out extra acidic juice that may give you a jabbing pain sooner or later. When you become depressed or fearful, your stomach lining turns pale and cuts down the juice supply. In sudden, acute stress such as an injury, the stomach is very likely to stop working entirely until the crisis is past; primitive body wisdom mobilizes energy for flight or fight.

The stomach's main job is, of course, food processing—mixing food with enzymes and breaking down proteins and fats. The powerful acid, mainly hydrochloric, in the stomach juice is there to assist the action of enzymes. As you know if you've ever vomited, the acid of gastric juice is so sharp that it can sear and damage tissues in the nose and throat, and even the stomach can be injured by its own juices when it develops an ulcer or is otherwise wounded.

Sweeping squeeze-waves travel from the top to the bottom of the stomach, moving its contents along into the duodenum, the receiving chamber for the intestine where nearly all the absorption of nutrients takes place. The entire food mass remains liquid throughout its trip through the small bowel. Later, in the colon, moisture is squeezed out, leaving a semisolid mass to be excreted.

From the beginning, the body has been adding dozens of different kinds of digestive juices to the foodstuff: saliva in the mouth, then stomach juices, then small-bowel juices, each kind spiked with special enzymes for breaking down specific food substances. Two glandular organs that lie in the neighborhood but outside the bowel itself —the liver and the pancreas—add their juices too. The gall bladder, storing bile to help handle fat globules, is a very useful receptacle when it's in good health, but it can safely be removed if it becomes diseased.

Absorption into the bloodstream through the delicate walls of tissue takes place all along the way. In the stomach itself not much gets absorbed but some fluids; most absorption goes on in the small intestine, which is lined with millions of tiny fingers, called villi, rich in blood vessels and in constant waving motion like tropical aquatic plans. Minerals as well as vitamins are absorbed through the intestinal walls. Protein, made up of amino acids, gets chopped down into its constituents once more. Carbohydrate, a big food molecule, gets cut down into glucose. Fat is changed into fatty acids and glycerol molecules.

Our own decisions about what we eat, how much we eat and how we manage the pressure of our daily lives can affect the working of the digestive system. (In chapters 2 and 4 you will find some pointers about digestion and indigestion.)

Reproductive System

Some women bear several children, many have one or two, and others never have any babies at all. Yet the possession of the genital and reproductive tract is a predominant fact of our existence, and during the thirty-five to forty years of childbearing capability we are continuously in one phase or another of reproductive functioning. The mystery and power of sexuality pervade the lives and behavior of both women and men, and our sense of our sex is closely bound with our sense of self.

The two ovaries—first station of the reproductive process—are elegant egg factories about the size of the tip of the thumb and oval in shape (literally, "egg-shaped"). Near each ovary the delicate Fallopian tubes open out in a funnel, a fimbriate structure as beautiful as a flower. As one ripened egg slips out of the left or the right ovary each month, it glides through the reaching funnel into the tube, where it either mates with a spermatozoon or breaks down and is

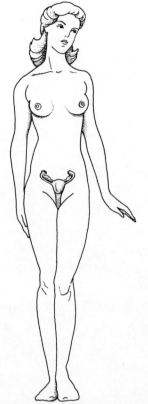

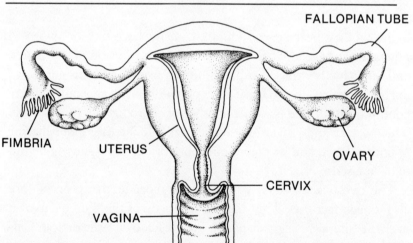

Typical woman in drawing (top) *shows approximate size and location of reproductive organs: Fallopian tubes, ovaries and uterus. Uterus may tilt forward, downward or back and still be normal. Enlarged cross section* (below) *shows tube fimbria ("fingers") in position to capture egg released from ovaries, and wedge-shaped uterine cavity.*

discarded along with the disposable uterine lining in the process we know as menstruation.

Simple? Anything but. Only the fact that most women experience this process, called ovulation, about 500 times during their lives makes it seem commonplace. Gynecologists sometimes remark that the more they study the intricacy and the delicate balance of the female reproductive system, the more awed and admiring they become.

The uterus, which is most often compared to a small pear (three inches long) hanging upside down within the shelter of the bony pelvic house, opens at its lower end in a cervix, or neck. With sexual mating, sperm cells race through the cervical opening into the

LIFE STAGES OF UTERUS SIZE

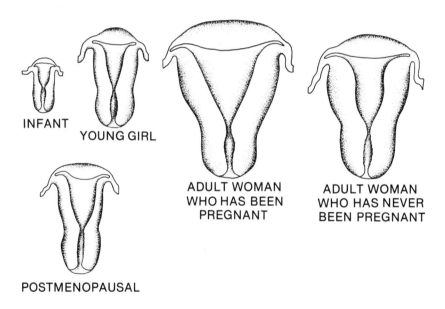

INFANT

YOUNG GIRL

ADULT WOMAN WHO HAS BEEN PREGNANT

ADULT WOMAN WHO HAS NEVER BEEN PREGNANT

POSTMENOPAUSAL

At birth, the uterus is slightly over one inch long. The "corpus," or body of the uterus, is about one-half the length of the cervix. After puberty, a woman who has never been pregnant will have a uterus between two and a half to three inches long; the corpus and cervix will be approximately equal in length. After childbearing, the uterus will reach three and a half inches in length; at this time the cervix will be half the length of the corpus. Following the menopause, the uterus will shrink somewhat due to decreased estrogen stimulation and may eventually become very small.

uterus and up the Fallopian tubes. There, fertilization of the egg takes place. The fertilized egg attaches itself to the inside of the uterus, where it proceeds to grow, incorporating characteristics of the man and woman who started it all. After approximately 40 weeks of development, the newborn leaves the mother's uterus, passes through the vaginal vault that is now a birth canal, and with considerable effort from both parties, emerges into the outside world.

Such normal female functions as pregnancy, childbirth and menstruation are fortunately no longer considered forms of sickness. Now that women have more control over their reproductive role, they need to replace some of the old mistaken attitudes that linked these functions with "sickness" and realize instead that the reproductive process is part of "wellness."

During the Victorian era, a woman could not have her body examined by a male doctor but had to point out on a figurine or a drawing where her pain was. Only another woman could give a woman direct physical care. Even in quite recent times, the sexual hush was so profound that women often did not know the names, or the existence, of their genital parts.

Today these veils have been lifted, thanks to increased knowledge and more open attitudes toward the role of sexual factors in our lives. Gynecologic health care and hygiene have brought benefits that were not anticipated even a generation ago. (In Part II we will discuss gynecologic problems in some detail.) A woman is certainly not just a reproductive machine as some old-fashioned males believed, but her reproductive equipment is so intricate and priceless that it behooves her to know it well and to care for it properly.

One Body, Many Systems

We have discussed briefly only a few of the body's systems, and even these are highly arbitrary divisions. They exist only to enable us to grasp the various functions of our physical selves. The systems influence and support one another—sometimes fairly independently, like the digestive process, which can be suspended for a while;

sometimes inextricably, as in the immediate dependence of the brain on the blood supply, and the dependence of circulation on direction from the brain-controlled nervous system.

In the remainder of this book we want to share with you a wide assortment of information, relating it to the best ideas that are now available for maintaining and enhancing your health and for handling problems if they arise.

2

GROUND RULES FOR HEALTH

Your Habits Can Be Your Best Friends

We are, in real life, a reasonably healthy people. Far from being ineptly put together, we are amazingly tough, durable organisms, full of health, ready for most contingencies.

—*Lewis Thomas,*
The Medusa and the Snail

Barring any unpreventable diseases and disabilities, the continuing state of our health is largely up to ourselves alone. It has been said that we ought to pay doctors for keeping us in health instead of treating us after we get sick. This is nonsense. Doctors can medicate, vaccinate and operate. They can advise and instruct. But they cannot live our lives for us or pursue a healthy lifestyle in our behalf. With medical care as a backup, it's the care we take of ourselves that counts.

The best approach to good self-care is through sound personal habits; forming useful ones, dropping useless or harmful ones. Developing excellent health habits can help you remain well without constant decision making, anxiety or conscious effort. Some of them, good and bad, that influence life, death and health include, for example, your *diet*. Virtually unlimited choices and amounts of food provide us freedom to develop anything from very good to very poor eating habits.

Evidence continues to pile up, proving that *cigarette smoking* is harmful in itself, and that it can make almost any other health problem worse.

The risks of *drinking* are still being measured. Current indications are that moderate intake of alcohol can be beneficial, but pregnant women, people who can't handle liquor, and those with various health problems should be cautious.

It is obviously wise to faithfully take *medication* prescribed for regulating a chronic condition like high blood pressure. But dependence on laxatives, aspirin, sleep aids and other such remedies should be avoided.

Now let's examine these habits more closely, as well as a range of other customs including exercise, dental habits, skin-care habits, bowel and bladder habits, sleep, posture and body hygiene.

Your Diet

Nutritionists are fond of saying that you are what you eat. It's a fearsome thought; but perhaps it's a good way to emphasize the importance of food preferences. A good diet delivers numerous benefits. It provides energy, rebuilds tissues, maintains biochemical balances, prevents certain diseases and is one of life's major pleasures.

For good health, eating should be based on nutritional values, not merely on efforts to cut down calories and control weight. Good nutrition guidebooks are available in bookstores to give you information on what nutrients are present in commonly used foods. Select one that provides authoritative charts showing the calorie, protein, carbohydrate and fat content of average food portions. Then look for vitamin and mineral content. The National Academy of Sciences publishes the very informative *Recommended Dietary Allowances,* which lists recommended daily amounts of all major vitamins and minerals for which requirements are recognized (along with calorie and protein needs) for infants, children, males, females, and pregnant and nursing women. This guide also explains what these nutrients are and how they work in the body.

Nutrition authorities insist that a wide variety of healthful foods in one's diet is necessary to provide ample insurance against vitamin or mineral deficiencies. It should be added, however, that more than half of the average American diet now consists of "processed" foods —which have been heat-treated, refined, preserved or put through other manufacturing steps likely to remove or destroy nutrient val-

NUTRIENTS: WHERE TO FIND THEM

Nutrient	Important Sources of Nutrient	What they do for you
Protein	Meat, poultry, fish, dried beans and peas, eggs, milk, cheese	Constitutes part of the structure of every cell such as muscle, blood, and bone; supports growth and maintains healthy body cells.
Vitamin A	Liver, carrots, sweet potatoes, greens, butter, margarine	Assists formation and maintenance of skin and mucous membranes that line the body cavities and tracts, such as nasal passages and intestinal tract, thus increasing resistance to infection.
Vitamin C	Broccoli, oranges, papaya, grapefruit, mango, strawberries	Forms cementing substances, such as collagen, that hold body cells together, thus strengthening blood vessels, hastening healing of wounds and bones and increasing resistance to infection.
Thiamin (B_1)	Lean pork, nuts, fortified cereal products	Aids in utilization of energy. Contributes to normal functioning of nervous system.
Riboflavin (B_2)	Liver, milk, yogurt, cottage cheese	Aids in utilization of energy. Promotes healthy skin and eyes.
Niacin	Liver, peanuts, meat, fish, poultry, fortified cereal products	Aids in utilization of energy. Aids digestion and fosters normal appetite.
Calcium	Milk, yogurt, cheese, sardines and salmon with bones, collard, kale, turnip and mustard greens	Combines with other minerals within a protein framework to give structure and strength to bones and teeth.
Iron	Enriched farina, red meat, prune juice, liver, dried beans and peas	Combines with protein to form hemoglobin, the red substance in blood that carries oxygen to and carbon dioxide from the cells. Prevents nutritional anemia and its accompanying fatigue. Increases resistance to infection.
Vitamin D	Vitamin D milk, fish, liver, oils, sunshine on skin (not a food)	Helps absorb calcium from the digestive tract and builds calcium and phosphorus into bone.
Vitamin E	Vegetable oils, green leafy vegetables, whole grain cereals, wheat germ, butter, egg yolk, milkfat	Protects vitamin A and unsaturated fatty acids from destruction by oxygen. Exact biochemical mechanism by which it functions still unknown.
Vitamin B_6	Beef, liver, pork, ham, lima beans, bananas, whole grain cereals	Assists in red blood cell regeneration. Helps regulate the use of protein, fat, and carbohydrate.

Nutrient	Important Sources of Nutrient	What they do for you
Folic Acid (Folacin)	Green leafy vegetables, liver, dry legumes, nuts, whole grain cereals, some fruits such as oranges	Assists in normal blood formation. Helps enzyme and other biochemical systems function.
Vitamin B_{12}	Only in animal foods—liver, meat, fish, shellfish, milk, milk products, eggs, poultry. Vegetarian diets should include milk or a B_{12} supplement	Assists in the maintenance of nerve tissues and normal blood formation.
Phosphorus	Milk and milk products, meat, poultry fish, eggs, whole grain cereals, legumes	Combines with calcium to give bones and teeth strength. Helps regulate many internal activities of the body.
Iodine	Seafoods, iodized salt	Helps regulate the rate at which the body uses energy.
Magnesium	Legumes, whole grain cereals, milk, meat, nuts, seafood, eggs, green vegetables	Helps regulate the use of carbohydrate and production of energy within the cells. Helps nerves and muscles work.
Zinc	Meat, liver, eggs, oysters, other seafoods, milk, whole grain cereals	Becomes part of several enzymes and insulin.

These vitamins and minerals can be obtained by eating a variety of foods from each of the four food groups. These are milk, meat, vegetable-fruit, and bread-cereal. By following this regimen you will be assured of receiving all the essential vitamins and minerals that your body needs to function properly.

RECOMMENDED DAILY DIETARY ALLOWANCES [a]

	Age (years)	Weight (lb)	Height (in)	Protein[1]	Fat-Soluble Vitamins			Water-Soluble Vitamins							Minerals					
					Vitamin A[2]	Vitamin D[2]	Vitamin E[3]	Vitamin C[3]	Thiamin[3]	Riboflavin[3]	Niacin[3]	Vitamin B-6[3]	Folacin[2]	Vitamin B-12[2]	Calcium[3]	Phosphorus[3]	Magnesium[3]	Iron[3]	Zinc[3]	Iodine[2]
Females	11-14	101	62	46	800	10	8	50	1.1	1.3	15	1.8	400	3.0	1200	1200	300	18	15	150
	15-18	120	64	46	800	10	8	60	1.1	1.3	14	2.0	400	3.0	1200	1200	300	18	15	150
	19-22	120	64	44	800	7.5	8	60	1.1	1.3	14	2.0	400	3.0	800	800	300	18	15	150
	23-50	120	64	44	800	5	8	60	1.0	1.2	13	2.0	400	3.0	800	800	300	18	15	150
	51+	120	64	44	800	5	8	60	1.0	1.2	13	2.0	400	3.0	800	800	300	10	15	150
Pregnant[c]				+30	+200	+5	+2	+20	+0.4	+0.3	+2	+0.6	+400	+1.0	+400	+400	+150	b	+5	+25
Lactating[c]				+20	+400	+5	+3	+40	+0.5	+0.5	+5	+0.5	+100	+1.0	+400	+400	+150	b	+10	+50

[a] The allowances are intended to provide for individual variations among most normal women as they live in the United States under usual environmental stresses. Diets should be based on a variety of common foods in order to provide other nutrients for which human requirements have been less well defined.

[b] The increased requirement during pregnancy cannot be met by the iron content of habitual American diets nor by the existing iron stores of many women; therefore the use of 30-60 mg of supplemental iron is recommended. Iron needs during lactation are not substantially different from those of nonpregnant women, but continued supplementation of the mother for 2-3 months after the baby's birth is advisable in order to replenish stores depleted by pregnancy.

[c] The plus signs signify the additional amounts of nutrients that a pregnant or lactating woman needs daily.

[1] grams

[2] micrograms

[3] milligrams

ues. Therefore, as we reach for the wide variety of foods, as suggested, it's best to reach in particular for a good proportion of unprocessed foods such as fresh vegetables, fruits, grains and nuts.

In this land of too much plenty, what we restrict in our diet may be as important as what we include. Taking a close look at the "average" diet, nutrition researchers tell us that our menus could best be improved by squeezing out, not putting in. If you eat as most Americans do, consider the following suggestions from the Surgeon General's report entitled *Healthy People:*

• Eat only enough calories to meet body needs and maintain desirable weight (which means fewer calories if you're overweight).

• Use less saturated fat and cholesterol-bearing foods. Animal fat, including butterfat in dairy foods, is highly saturated. Red meat, eggs and most seafoods are high in cholesterol, which helps to form fatty globules called lipoproteins.

• Use less salt. This actually means less sodium, of which common table salt is the most prominent example. Experts say that the body's actual need for salt amounts to only about one gram (one-fifth teaspoonful) daily, but Americans commonly use as much as fifteen times that amount. People who already have high blood pressure are advised to reduce their salt intake, but it's also believed that cutting down salt may actually help to prevent the development of high blood pressure.

• Use less sugar. Since sugar supplies calories without any redeeming nutritional value, and since sugar is blamed for a good deal of tooth decay, it's safe to bet that most of us eat far too much of it. Per capita consumption of sugar and sweeteners amounts to more than 125 pounds per year. This represents 20 percent of the average American's total calorie intake, so it appears that the necessary vitamins, minerals and other nutrients must be obtained from the remaining 80 percent of the diet.

Unlike starch, a complex carbohydrate, sugar is a simple carbohydrate. Its most common form is sucrose, or regular table sugar. This disaccharide, or double sugar, is formed of a molecule of glucose and a molecule of fructose. Glucose is the predominating sugar circulating in the blood; fructose means fruit sugar, though the sugar in fruit is really only 20 to 40 percent fructose.

As this is written, we are witnessing a surge of popularity for powdered fructose, along with claims of its effectiveness in weight-loss diets. Other claims, that fructose is more "natural" than other forms of sugar, are not borne out by chemical fact. Fructose is, in fact, manufactured by splitting the fructose molecule from ordinary sucrose, cane or beet sugar. Liquid fructose (actually a high fructose syrup) is made from corn syrup treated with enzymes to convert part of its glucose to fructose. Contrary to some advertising claims, fructose is even more processed, more "refined," than regular white granulated sugar—and just as empty of nutrients, except for calories.

The Surgeon General's report, reflecting wide-scale nutrition studies, recommends increased use of complex carbohydrates, or starches, occurring in whole grains, fruits and vegetables. This means replacing part of the calories obtained from fats and protein with foods like bread, potatoes, beans, peas, rice and other grains. An added benefit of this diet change would be an increase in fiber, or bulk. To reduce your caloric intake, use more fish, poultry, legumes or beans as protein sources, and less red meat.

Women may have special nutritional needs at certain times, either because of heavy menstrual flow, use of the pill or pregnancy. A simple blood count can indicate whether you need supplemental iron to replace the loss during menstruation. But excess ingested iron can cause abdominal cramps and can be toxic. The pill may also increase the need for vitamin B_6 and folate (another B vitamin), as does pregnancy. Many physicians will point out that a nutritious diet will provide adequate amounts of these vitamins, but for those of us who know how often we fail to eat properly, taking vitamin supplements with folate and B_6 while on the pill or during pregnancy may be a good idea. Calcium supplementation may also be needed in pregnancy, and particularly in breast-feeding. (See Chapter 6 for more details.)

What are our health payoffs for changes in our eating habits? Better general health, certainly. Control of weight, too; just trimming excess fat and sugar from the diet tends to correct a too high calorie level. Diabetes is rare in countries that have a low incidence of obesity and low sugar consumption. It is common in countries such as the United States, where obesity and overuse of sugar are prevalent. Finally, evidence is building that a prudent diet may offer protection against some cancers. Studies of populations throughout the world provide clues that too much animal protein—red meat in particular—may be linked to colon and breast cancer, as is too little plant fiber and too much fat. At this time, further studies are being made, reaching for clearer findings to guide us in forming the best possible eating habits.

Your Exercise Program

In recent years Americans by the millions have taken to the road-ways and running paths. Greatly increased, too, are the numbers of people taking part in racquet sports, swimming, and cross-country skiing. Although the steadily falling death rate from heart attacks may be attributed to a number of factors, one of them is certainly America's interest in exercise.

Most of us probably exercise for the sense of well-being it gives us, some of us simply because it's fun. When physical activity is adequate, it increases body strength and endurance, improves and preserves flexibility, and adds to attractiveness. For many people, a valued benefit is relief from stress and anxiety.

Does exercise really help you avoid overweight? There's a prevail-ing notion that in order to burn up the 3,600 calories in a pound of fat, you'd have to exercise violently and constantly for three days or so—and that, furthermore, your appetite would increase so much that you'd eat more food and thus negate the benefits of the exercise. This is myth and nonsense. According to a renowned nutrition authority, Jean Mayer, Ph.D., exercise will indeed help to control weight. For example, says Dr. Mayer, cross-country skiing over hard, level terrain at about 4 miles an hour burns up 600 calories an hour—and going uphill at maximum speed expends twice that amount, or 1,200 calories per hour. A half-hour of handball or squash each day, adds Dr. Mayer, means shedding sixteen pounds of fat per year.

Moreover, though physical activity does cause some appetite increase, food demand levels off as activity becomes really strenuous. And people with very low activity don't lower their appetites to match; with a continuing decline in action, the appetite may even rise slightly. So exercise is a must if your problem is keeping your weight down.

If you enjoy running, walking or swimming, you probably have a regular work-out schedule already. If you are inactive, or not active enough, you may be wondering how to get yourself on a program you can stick to and benefit from. Here are some suggestions:

• *The Total Woman's Fitness Guide,* by Gail Shierman, Ph.D., and Christine Haycock, M.D., for the nonathletic woman, gives exercises for strength, endurance and flexibility, all shown in photographs. You'll also get directions for measuring your fitness progress and checking pulse response to exertion.

• *Adult Physical Fitness,* a government publication from the President's Council on Physical Fitness, gives graded exercises geared to several levels of conditioning. The program includes warm-up exercises and tests that measure your fitness progress. This publication can be ordered from the U.S. Government Printing Office, Washington, D.C. 20402.

• Health clubs, as you'll see in the Yellow Pages of your telephone directory, offer a wide variety of facilities, services and classes. Some specialize in weight-loss programs only. Before you invest in a course or program at a commercial health club, go there, look the place over and watch how it operates. Make certain that large exercising apparatuses are under constant, trained supervision when being used by club patrons.

• Swimming pools and gymnasium facilities may be available at your local YWCA, YWHA or, at scheduled times, at the men's counterpart associations, the YMCA and the YMHA.

• High schools and junior and community colleges often make swimming-pool time available to residents during early morning or evening hours when the pool is not being used by the school.

• Skating rinks, both ice and roller, usually have courses of instruction.

• Many dance studios offer dance-exercise courses.

• Bicycle rental firms can usually be found near public bike paths. Along waterways you'll find canoes, rowboats, kayaks and racing shells for rent, and instructors to train you in using them safely and effectively. Tennis clubs and softball teams are available almost everywhere.

In short, there's a lot of action out there, yours if you wish to join it. You can also do a lot to keep fit all by yourself at home, with calisthenics and fitness exercises.

Sleep

In spite of the old eight-hours rule most of us were given in childhood, sleep requirements are highly individual and may range from as little as six hours to as much as ten hours a night. The best sleep rule for fitness is to develop a sleeping habit: bedtime approximately the same each night, rising time the same each morning. If you're not getting enough sleep, you probably will be aware of it. You'll be tired during the day or getting sleepy at inappropriate times. If you're sleeping too long, you may have problems with insomnia or growing lethargy in following days. (See Chapter 4 for insomnia problems.) If you have no health problems that interfere with sleep, your best bet is to form the habits that agree with you and stick to them as much as possible.

Body Care

• Care of the teeth, vital to health and fitness, should be a regular daily habit. Dental hygienists recommend a teeth-cleaning routine that includes thorough dental flossing of all between-teeth spaces, followed by several minutes of brushing and gum massage.
• Care of your skin is more than a beauty habit. The skin is an organ weighing about twenty-five pounds, with important work to do in moving wastes and maintaining body temperature. It tends to take care of itself very well, but it may signal by eruptions, color changes and other signs when something is physically wrong. It's important to protect the skin against excess sun exposure, both to avoid premature aging and to prevent actinic, or sun-caused, skin

cancers. Sunscreen lotions come in a number of strengths and are very effective in preventing exposure of the skin to ultraviolet rays and in limiting the tanning effect. High concentrations protect extremely light and delicate skin; lesser concentrations protect darker skins and permit moderate suntanning. For skin health in sunny seasons, using a sunscreen is a recommended habit. The recent fad of "tanning parlors" is almost universally condemned by skin experts. The high levels of ultraviolet exposure used to promote "instant tans" are known to be carcinogenic. When balanced against the premature aging of the skin and the increased risk of skin cancer incurred by deep tanning, a brief period of looking "fashionable" is a macabre price to pay.

• Good bowel and bladder habits are essential, both for fitness and for preventing eventual chronic disease conditions. (See Chapter 4 for constipation, which can result from faulty habits.)After ensuring proper diet and fluid intake, the most important habit is prompt attention to excretion signals. Urinating habits in particular affect your susceptibility to cystitis, the painful urinary-tract infection that becomes chronic in many women. One study showed that a high proportion of women who had repeated cystitis also had bad bladder-emptying habits. They tended to postpone urinating for one to six hours after the time-to-go signal. They also tended not to empty bladders promptly after sexual intercourse. Those who agreed to a regular regimen for urination were rewarded by a high rate of cleared-up urinary symptoms. Adequate fluid intake (six to eight glasses of water a day) is also important in preventing urinary-tract infections.

• Frequent vaginal douching is a questionable habit. It can shrink the tissues, make intercourse painful and cause vaginal irritation. Some women feel more comfortable if they douche occasionally, even though many gynecologists say douching isn't necessary at all. The operative word should be "moderation." The vaginal vault acts to cleanse itself by mucus secretion, which moves from the upper part down toward the entrance. Gentle cleansing in a bath or shower is recommended, using fingers and mild soapy water inside the lower two or three inches of the vagina. Perfumed spray or deodorant products for vaginal use are not generally recommended by gynecologists because of the risk of painful inflammation.

• Good posture can help you avoid muscle and skeletal strains and improve blood circulation. If your work involves standing for long hours, make a habit of elevating the legs at every rest opportunity. Exercise, weight control and support hose will help prevent varicose veins. Standing up for long periods can also be relieved by placing one foot on a low platform, such as a telephone book, alternating to the other foot from time to time. Brief limbering exercises, such as a stretching and reaching or neck rotation, can relieve tense muscles.

Bad Habits

• As you'll read elsewhere in this book, cigarette smoking is one habit with absolutely nothing to recommend it as far as health is concerned. Besides being a threat to heart function, increasing risk of lung cancer and other lung disease, smoking literally ages lung tissues. Medical authorities warn against smoking particularly during pregnancy because of the increased incidence of infants with low birth weight and greatly compromised health status who are born to smoking mothers. Most people with an established smoking habit find quitting difficult, and many need help from stop-smoking clinics and organizations. Your physician, too, can offer support and medication to help you through the withdrawal stages.

• Alcoholism is a major national problem. Women often fail to admit to themselves that they are dependent on alcohol before it is too late. If you find yourself "needing" a drink, drinking alone or getting into trouble because of drinking, obtain counseling before it becomes a crippling habit. Groups such as Alcoholics Anonymous have kept millions of susceptible people away from alcohol. Recently it has been established that even moderate use of alcohol during pregnancy can greatly increase the risk of birth defects. The fetus is especially vulnerable in very early stages, when many women are not yet aware they are pregnant. It's a good idea, therefore, to abstain completely from alcohol, even beer and wine, when you are planning to become pregnant.

For nonpregnant women, doctors have found that one or two drinks daily may lower heart-attack rates as compared to the incidence among total abstainers. This suggests the conclusion that a very modest happy hour may actually be good for you—pleasant news indeed. Many physicians have been put in a quandary by this information, since alcoholism is a problem of immense proportions here and in other countries, and any medical approval of drinking could serve as a go-ahead for many alcoholics, who usually are unable to drink moderately. In ordinary circumstances the best bottom line is that a drink should be a special treat, not a habit. Also, don't forget that when used with some medications, alcohol can cause death by changing or greatly increasing the drug's effect. Therefore, when a drug is being prescribed for you, it's a good idea to ask about its interactions with alcohol. This easily accessible information could save you from needless harm or even tragedy.

• Drugs are another major national problem. Although there is little evidence that occasional marijuana use is more damaging than moderate alcohol use, the dangers of addictive drugs and the abuse of street drugs are all too apparent to most sensible people. Probably more serious in terms of the general population are the more insidious dangers of abuse of common prescription and over-the-counter "medications." Too many women become addicted to "uppers" for their diets and "downers" for their nerves, and at times doctors may find it easier to write a tranquilizer prescription than to explore the reasons why a woman's "nerves" are bothering her. Diet pills are not the answer to obesity—dieting is. Minor tranquilizers are not the answer to "nerves"—learning to cope with stress in a meaningful fashion is. There is nothing intrinsically harmful in the occasional use of an appetite suppressant or minor tranquilizer, but the dangers of chronic abuse are overwhelming. Chronic use is addictive and can destroy your normal coping mechanisms. And, finally, any drug taken frequently by women will eventually be used by women in early stages of pregnancy and potentially endanger the developing baby.

It is ironic that in a nation which has all but eliminated the natural scourges of plague, polio, tuberculosis and other diseases that destroyed our ancestors, we have replaced them with man-made scourges that destroy us: smoking, obesity, alcoholism. Nothing can guarantee you a healthy body, but with proper habits you can avoid double-crossing the one you have.

3

YOU AND YOUR DOCTOR

How do you go about finding the best doctor for you? Even if you read the scores of articles and books giving advice on the subject, the process of selecting a personal physician is something like dating by computer, with many facts and bits of data in place but with the chemistry of personalities still to be resolved.

There are, however, valuable guidelines both for selecting and for working with a physician. In the following pages we will discuss the basic steps you can take to learn how the doctor you're considering has been trained, the specialty qualifications he or she has received, his or her professional achievements, and the hospitals in which the doctor may practice. You'll want to know just what kinds of medical services the physician provides, and you should also know how to use your second-opinion option, should the occasion arise.

We will limit the discussion here to two kinds of doctors—the one for general health care, who may be a general practice, family practice or internal medicine physician; and the gynecologist or gynecologist-obstetrician. Many women have no regular physician besides their gynecologist; it is best to also have a generalist of one of the three groups named above. Your whole body, not just your reproductive system, deserves medical attention.

If you are new to an area, and you want to get established with a physician close at hand, you may take one of these approaches: See the "Physicians and Surgeons" listing in the Yellow Pages of your telephone book, or call your county medical association or the local, or city, medical society. These organizations will give you the names of doctors near you, but they will not recommend any specific individual. The choice is yours.

Perhaps the most thorough procedure is to go to your public library and ask to see the *Directory of Medical Specialists* and the *American Medical Directory*. The *Directory of Medical Specialists* gives information on physicians who are "board-certified" specialists, thus enabling you to find information on those in family practice, which is a specialty, internal medicine, and of course gynecology. The *American Medical Directory*, on the other hand, includes all doctors, board-certified or not, who belong to the American Medical Association. Both books are arranged geographically, so you can select doctors in your area. Both books give a good deal of information on each listed physician. You can learn the doctor's year of birth, medical school graduation, and licensing. You can also learn the doctor's first and second specialties, if any, and the date of specialty certification.

"Board-certified" means that a doctor has completed a period of practice, or residency, in a special area of medicine, and has passed the rigorous examinations of the professional board, or college, of that specialty. Board-eligible physicians will have completed their residencies, and most likely are in line for their board examinations after a required time. Board certification is not absolute proof that a particular doctor is the right one for you to consult, nor does lack of certification mean that a doctor is not competent. Certification does, however, indicate that the doctor has had extra specialized training and possesses a high level of competence, as tested by fellow physicians in that specialty.

In practice, many people find a doctor by "word of mouth," by asking neighbors or friends. Often the best advertising a physician can have is a satisfied patient. A medical professional such as a nurse employed in a local hospital may be a good source of information. Also, local hospitals will provide names of physicians on their staffs who are willing to accept new patients.

Questions You Ask

When you call to make your initial appointment with a new doctor, you can get answers to several important questions from the physician's appointment secretary. Following is a check list of such questions. You probably won't need to ask all of them; check those that apply to your needs, and don't hesitate to ask about anything you want to know. Almost all doctors say they welcome patients' questions and willingly answer them. First port-of-call, however, should be the physician's secretary; answering questions is part of her job.

1. What are the doctor's basic fees, and what is included? For example, if laboratory tests are done, are they billed separately?

2. Does the doctor do a general physical examination? If you don't have a separate gynecologist, does this doctor do a Pap smear, pelvic examination, VD tests? Some internists, not all, do pelvic examinations (an internal examination of the genital tract). Not all gynecologists perform obstetrics; this can be important if you're pregnant or planning to have a baby.

3. Does the doctor provide contraceptive counsel? Does he prescribe the pill, insert IUDs, fit diaphragms? Does the physician perform abortions? Sterilizations?

4. At what hospitals does the doctor have staff privileges? It may be important to know whether your doctor can care for you in a hospital near your home (although some very good physicians confine themselves to office practice and refer to colleagues any patients who need hospital care). How large is the hospital? Does the doctor have a teaching appointment at a hospital associated with a medical school? This is one sign that the doctor is prominent in a specialty and up to date in medical advances.

5. Is the doctor in a group practice? An advantage might be that another doctor in the group would be available to you when your physician is away. On the other hand, you may feel you don't have a guarantee of as much access to your own physician in a group-practice setting as you might wish.

6. If the doctor is in solo practice, ask whether other doctors cover calls when he or she is not available.

7. What is the doctor's payment policy? Some send statements; others prefer payment at each visit. Clinics and large group practices may bill your medical insurance company and then bill you later for any items not covered by your insurance. You should not expect, however, a physician in private practice to handle billing this way; to do so would add considerably to the physician's cost of running his office.

8. If it's applicable in your case, does the doctor accept Medicare or Medicaid patients?

9. Does the doctor make house calls? Also, in an emergency or disabling illness, where can you get prompt medical care?

Questions the Doctor Asks

The physician or assistant will want to take your medical history, as you know if you've ever consulted a doctor. It's a highly important document that helps the doctor to evaluate any problems you have and to carry on your continuing care. Answer all questions as completely as possible. Some doctors update the medical history every year or so, adding any events that may have occurred in the meantime, such as the death or serious illness of a family member, which could influence or provide clues to your own health risks. With a new doctor, offer the name and address of your previous physician so your past medical record can be requested.

1. You'll be asked about your general health, your health in childhood, and any illnesses, surgery, hospitalizations, injuries and childbirth.

2. You may be asked about health problems of your close relatives, living or dead. Such ailments include anemia, allergies, arthritis, abnormal bleeding, cancer, diabetes, endocrine diseases, epilepsy, gout, heart disease, high blood pressure, jaundice, kidney disease, mental retardation, migraine, obesity, psychiatric illness and tuberculosis.

3. You may be asked about specific organs or body systems. Some examples are: breathing problems, coughs, bleeding problems, digestive trouble, insomnia, menstrual problems.

4. Don't be surprised if the physician asks specific questions about your present lifestyle: your job, living situation, activities, personal habits and sex life. The doctor is not being personally inquisitive—these are vital factors in your overall health picture and can be important to the doctor in correctly analyzing your symptoms or detecting diseases you may have.

5. Finally, if you have come not for just a checkup, your doctor will need to know all about the symptoms or illness you are having now.

The most effective way you can take part in this discussion is to prepare notes in advance. You'd be surprised at the things you'll forget when you're in the doctor's office. Among the items to list are your symptoms—all of them, and how long and how often you've had them; *all* medications you take, either regularly or frequently, including oral contraceptives, aspirin, sleeping pills, vitamins, laxatives, tranquilizers. List your allergies, particularly allergies to drugs such as penicillin. Think back and write down your past illnesses and hospitalizations and their dates. When you go to see the doctor, take along your immunization record if possible.

Before you go for your appointment, it's a good idea to reread your health-insurance policy, with special attention to what's included and excluded.

What to Expect

You should not be embarrassed to ask the doctor any question at all regarding your body or your health. Be assured that you are not going to surprise, shock or elicit disapproval from any doctor you'd want to continue consulting. If you feel inhibited, make a special effort to bring out your concerns about pain, emotional distress and fears. Don't merely ask for a checkup when you really want to know if you have VD or cancer. Leveling with your physician can be essential to your health.

In return, your physician can be expected to answer, not avoid, your questions. This includes explanation of the diagnosis, the treatment proposed and the prescribed medication. But you should ask the questions; don't expect the doctor to volunteer a fully detailed explanation. There are many patients who want only to be given directions, not full explanations, and doctors must take that into account. So if you want complete answers, ask questions. Taking down notes helps you to be sure you have understood and have your directions straight. Studies show that time after time, patients hear what the doctor says "selectively"—that is, the memory blocks out things the patient doesn't wish to hear or doesn't understand clearly.

The physician keeps a file on each patient. This medical record contains your original medical history and an ongoing account of each visit you make. It also contains medicines prescribed, your symptoms, your weight, blood pressure and the results of any tests that are given to you. By keeping these records, the doctor avoids having to entrust to memory the details of your physical condition.

Even though these records are about you, they belong to the physician. Sometimes patients fear that the doctor is not telling them everything he is putting in the medical record, and in certain instances this may be true. For example, the doctor may have made notes of a clinical impression, or an opinion on a possible diagnosis that is not yet borne out by actual tests. The doctor may do this as a simple reminder to himself to check out the condition the next time he sees you. Doctors' records can be subpoenaed (that is, taken into court in a lawsuit), so there is every reason for them to be a full and candid account of a patient's condition and treatment.

Many practicing doctors will resist turning over the entire medical record to a patient. Among the reasons for this is the fact that many of the notes are written in semi-illegible handwriting and in a medical jargon, or shorthand, which can easily be misunderstood and misinterpreted by a nonmedical person. Other physicians, however, are willing to share medical records with their patients.

You may wish to keep your own medical record, or diary, by taking notes at each office visit, asking the doctor for test and examination results, including pulse rate and blood pressure, and adding instructions and medications received from the physician. If you feel something is wrong with your medical care or that important information is being withheld from you, you have a legal right to ask your lawyer to request your medical records.

You should also be aware that agencies such as government auditors or insurance carriers often request information from your medical records. Unfortunately, the days of complete privacy vanished with the arrival of third-party payments for medical care. Generally, medical information will be made available only when you have specifically and in writing approved its release, but if you are concerned about confidentiality, it is reasonable to ask your physician about this issue. As a rule, private physicians' records will be more confidential than will clinic notes or hospital records, which a larger number of personnel will have access to. Psychiatric records are generally well protected; in many hospitals, psychiatric records are kept separately from general medical records.

If you change from one doctor to another, you may ask your former physician to relay your medical record to your new one. This may prevent considerable retesting and can give your new doctor important background on your past illnesses and treatments. Physicians say they feel that it's a professional obligation to supply patients' records to new physicians requesting them—provided, of course, that the patient makes the request. Such a report should add up to better medical care for you.

More Things to Learn from Your Doctor

When you receive a prescription from your doctor, look at it while the physician repeats the instructions for taking the medicine. The letters "b.i.d.," "t.i.d." and "q.i.d" are merely shorthand Latin for telling you how often each day—twice, three times, four times— you're to take the medicine. The pharmacist will type them in English on the prescription label. Your doctor is likely to prescribe the drug by its brand name, but it may also be written in its generic form—meaning that the basic medication can be formulated by any number of pharmaceutical manufacturers, often at a considerable reduction in cost. Some states require prescription forms to carry a space for the generic name of a drug, but if your state does not, always ask your doctor to let you know what the name is.

Ask your doctor whether you should continue taking the medicine until the entire prescription is used up. This is very important with antibiotics, for example, where stopping the doses when you feel better or symptoms go away may bring on a relapse, or worse, may allow the disease organism to develop resistance to drugs. Other medicines, such as painkillers and cough medications, may be prescribed to be taken as needed. Be sure the instructions are clear about spacing the doses when they simply say "Take as needed."

Information leaflets—sometimes called package inserts—are being required by law for more and more medications, notably for oral contraceptives and estrogen preparations. If your doctor gives you some such medication in the office to tide you over until a prescription is filled, you will also be given any required information in leaflet form. The pharmacist will hand you the leaflet when you receive the prescription.

Read these materials carefully, even though they are in fine print and may even seem somewhat alarming. They tell all about side effects, possible harmful results in susceptible people, and contraindications, which means conditions in which the drug should not be used. Ask your physician about anything in this material that you don't understand or that worries you.

For some medical and surgical procedures, the doctor is required by law to obtain your *informed consent.* This means that the physician must explain any possible risks to you which might result from the treatment, and must see that you understand what is being done. This is a valuable protection for you, helps you to take part in your own health care, and reinforces the working relationship between you and your doctor. At one time, patients could be treated without understanding what was being done and without an opportunity to refuse treatment if they wished.

Your signature on the consent form is *not* a legal clearance for the doctor in case something goes wrong. The doctor's benefits from informed patient consent include knowing that the patient understands the treatment and has trust and confidence in it.

When you face a procedure or treatment that requires informed consent, you should take notes if possible. Also, if at all possible, have a family member or your closest friend present during the physician's explanation, to reinforce your understanding.

4

HOW DO YOU FEEL? WHAT SHOULD YOU DO?

It came out that illness of any sort was considered in Erewhon to be highly criminal and immoral; and that I was liable, even for catching cold, to be had up before the magistrates and imprisoned for a considerable period.

—*Samuel Butler,* Erewhon

When you feel generally awful but can't tell what's wrong, or when you have a definite symptom, pain or problem, it's important to identify the trouble at least enough to come to a decision on what course of action to take. Some people endure disorders that could be relieved by medical treatment; others consult their doctors repeatedly for illness and symptoms for which the physician honestly cannot find a medical cause. Such persons usually are not faking or imagining their illness, and they tend to go from doctor to doctor in search of relief.

In this chapter we will discuss some common pains and symptoms, and what they may be trying to tell you. Our goal is to give you some useful guidelines that will send you to a doctor when you do need medical attention and help you recognize and manage some other problems when self-understanding and care are all that is really required.

The "complaints" we'll talk about are usually not severe ones, though some of them, in some situations, could indicate serious conditions. Unfortunately, many are widely considered "women's problems." There is an underlying reason for this. Studies show that women consult physicians more readily than men do. This does not mean women go to doctors unnecessarily—it could mean instead that men often don't seek medical care when they should.

The "female" symptoms affect the various body systems and may arise at various ages. (See Chapter 11 for strictly gynecologic conditions.)

The Somatization Trap

There was a time when it was acceptable, even fashionable, for ladies to be delicate, weak and dizzy, to "swoon," "to faint dead away." Near-lethal corseting, deplorable health habits and society's expectations could account for much of this, and on occasion it probably rescued many a belle from an awkward encounter.

Also, in earlier days and to some extent in our own time, a good wife was supposed to be sexually available whenever her husband wished. To say "I really don't want to tonight" was unacceptable, but "I have a headache" was an adequate excuse.

Today, both men and women frequently "call in sick" on a job that is boring or disagreeable, and they may actually feel sick. Chances are they're "somatizing" an emotional problem. *Soma* means body, and to somatize is to shift the problem to the body. Instead of tackling the task of changing the working conditions or finding a new job, these people express their distress in the form of pain, digestive upset, a breathing problem or disturbed sleep. The pains and symptoms are very real and in time may lead to disease. They're difficult to relieve because they reflect problems that can be solved only when confronted and dealt with directly.

Fatigue

The state of being continuously tired is an insidious problem. One tends to drag on and on, to "get used to it," and too often, do nothing about it. If you feel weary, and the condition has been going on for some time, take steps to find out what's wrong.

Disease conditions that can cause chronic fatigue include hypothyroidism (low thyroid function), hyperthyroidism (overactive thyroid), anemia, poor nutrition (overweight or underweight), flu and various viral infections, and, very rarely, mononucleosis, hepatitis or leukemia. These possible organic causes of fatigue, however, account for only a small percentage of cases. It is more likely that something in the daily habits needs to be adjusted.

Overwork, depression, poor sleeping habits or poor exercise patterns can cause chronic fatigue. A typical case in point is the overworked wife and mother whose family does not recognize she's putting in long, strenuous days, seven days a week, without time off for relaxation. Usually she doesn't realize herself that she's suffering from simple overwork; she wonders what's wrong with her.

One woman physician, for example, recalls when she was a medical student: "I went through a period of exhaustion, as many do. I slept poorly, didn't exercise, survived on peanut-butter sandwiches. I knew better, too. Eventually I broke the cycle by making a point of swimming or running every day and working as a waitress two evenings a week. The job gave me hard physical work and square meals while working, as well as enough pocket money to eat properly. I also got a needed break in the routine of constant study. Being physically tired at night solved all my sleeping problems."

Another frequent victim of fatigue is the would-be superwoman. This overachiever is usually a high-powered career woman. Typically, she puts in a long, hard office day followed by a long ride home. She cooks dinner, throws in a load of laundry, cleans up the house, spends some time with her children—and collapses just when her husband starts feeling romantic, having been relaxing with a drink and a newspaper since the end of his office day.

This problem has several clear solutions: Your husband can share the domestic workload. Housework can be streamlined to be less burdensome. Help can be hired. Or you can cut down your job hours. Whatever the chosen solution, the important first step is to recognize the source of fatigue and the need to deal with it.

Failing to eat properly and exercise regularly can produce chronic fatigue. These derelictions happen to women at every age, but young women are particularly susceptible. One physician who sees many patients with chronic fatigue cites this typical case:

"She was twenty-eight and three months pregnant. Her three

children were five, four, and two years old. She did all the housework and took care of the children alone. Her husband was becoming tense and hostile because she never felt like having sexual intercourse. Add it all up: three little children, another on the way, a house to manage without help, and an unsympathetic husband—and she wondered why she was so tired! It was quite likely, too, that her turned-off sexual feelings stemmed from the psychological association of intercourse with many children.

"At my suggestion, she brought her husband to the office. We discussed the enormous workload she was carrying and worked out ideas for rearranging her day, with a teen-age helper and some assistance from the children's grandmother, to allow an occasional bit of rest and relaxation. It helped immensely, of course. In many cases like this one, fatigue is the normal response to overwork instead of a symptom of disease. But it can certainly turn into a medical condition if it goes on for too long a time."

If you feel chronically tired, take a close look at your lifestyle. Are you bored, overworked, do you have poor health habits?

Suppose you organize your living pattern to allow for enough rest, a proper diet and adequate exercise, and you still continue to feel tired. Then you should have a medical evaluation. This may start with a general physical examination that may yield some clues for the physician. A blood count may detect or rule out anemia. Other tests include liver-function tests, thyroid tests and specific viral tests.

Remember, medical illness can trigger depression and poor appetite and failure to develop adequate exercise patterns, as well as the other way round. Most cases of chronic fatigue are related to lifestyle. Lifestyle faults plus medical illness may underlie fatigue.

Headaches

Most of us have had occasional, transient headaches from some specific cause. Common headache causes are stress (either physical or psychological pressure), blood-vessel constriction or dilation, muscular aches in the neck or jaw, food sensitivity, poorly fitted glasses, stuffy sinuses from allergy or infection, insufficient or disrupted sleep or high blood pressure.

Stress or sinus headaches can usually be relieved by aspirin or aspirin substitutes or, in case of allergy, by decongestants and antihistamines. Additional sleep often helps. People with liver trouble should avoid acetaminophen (aspirin substitute); people with stomach ulcers, asthma or digestive problems should avoid aspirin.

Migraine headache, as its sufferers know, is an intense, throbbing, usually one-sided pain that may be preceded by dizziness, blurred vision, face and hand numbness, and it may lead to nausea and vomiting. Each case of migraine needs individual medical evaluation and management because medications that help one migraine patient may not help another. Migraine tends to run in families, and though actual causes are not clear, victims usually discover and learn to avoid things that may trigger an attack, such as certain foods and drinks, situations involving bright lights, loud music or other sensory events. Migraine is often a premenstrual event.

On rare occasions, headache can be the major symptom of a serious condition. Among these conditions are brain or spinal-cord tumors, increased pressure within the brain or spinal cord, stroke or concussion. Danger signals calling for medical attention include deep, dull, steady pain that occurs regularly in the morning; blurred vision, facial paralysis or numbness and vomiting. Some of these symptoms also occur with migraine headaches and should be investigated in people with no migraine history. Any frequent severe headache that isn't relieved by simple medications should also be medically investigated.

Insomnia

> No small art it is to sleep: it is necessary for that
> purpose to keep awake all day.
>
> —*Friedrich Nietzsche,*
> Thus Spake Zarathustra

Difficulty in falling asleep or staying asleep is an age-old universal problem that is probably here to stay as long as there is human life. All of us have occasional bouts of insomnia; about a third of us often enough to consider it a problem.

Insomnia may have an organic or medical cause. It's likely to be severe pain, a constant cough or an irritable bowel that keeps you awake for obvious reasons. But by far the most frequent causes of insomnia are stress, nervousness, worry, not enough daytime activity, or something in your daily actions that you probably can correct.

To get adequate rest you need to go through the four stages of the sleep cycle, usually several times during the night. As you fall asleep your body temperature drops and the brain activity known as "alpha rhythm" waves begins. Your heartbeat slows down and your muscles relax. Stage two features high brain-wave activity, which becomes slow and sweeping in stage three. You're relaxed and breathing evenly. Stage four is deep sleep, with the brain registering delta waves. After only a few minutes of this you rise almost to awakening and go into REM (rapid eye movement) sleep, the stage at which you most often dream. Then you'll most likely slip back to stage two and start the cycle again.

Scientists who uncovered the physiology of sleep also found that people deprived of any one of the stages became upset. Without REM sleep one becomes nervous and irritable, while deprivation of delta-wave sleep produces depression. Since drugs and sedatives may block off one or more of the sleep stages, their side effects can be quite harmful.

Following are some suggestions for getting a good solid night's rest. If you have a simple sleep problem, these tips should help you. If you have a severe or disabling sleep problem that interferes with your daytime activity, you should see a physician who will explore all the possible medical causes. He may even refer you to a specialist for further examination.

• Establish regular sleeping hours. Get up at the same time each day and retire near the same hour each night.
• Avoid stimulants—coffee, tea, cola drinks, diet pills that contain amphetamines.
• Have your evening meal several hours before bedtime. You may also need to give up dinnertime coffee or tea.
• For some people, warm or cold milk or hot chocolate is helpful. Milk contains tryptophan, an amino acid found to have an effect on brain hormones that induce sleep.

• Relax before bedtime with music, television or light reading.

• Be sure your bedroom is a place of peace—quiet, dark and restful. Don't conduct business or do homework from your bed; it's hard to forget when you turn off the light. If you're sensitive to disturbance, don't hesitate to use a sleeping mask or ear plugs.

• Do not nap. Many people who complain about insomnia allow themselves to doze off during the day. (Some high-powered people claim to subsist on catnaps, but they don't suffer from insomnia.)

• If you absolutely cannot sleep, get out of bed and do something that engrosses you until you simply feel ready for bed. Many people just don't need as much sleep as they think they do.

Prescription drugs are taken for insomnia. In addition, Americans spend about $25 million each year for over-the-counter sleep medicines. Extensive research and government review have found that many of these drugs either don't work or are unsafe. Those medicines that are considered effective usually contain antihistamine, an ingredient that can make one drowsy. The federal Food and Drug Administration removed a great many nonprescription sleep drugs from the market in 1979 after finding that their main ingredient, the antihistamine methapyrilene, was cancer-causing in animal tests. Many of the sleep aids have been reformulated and are back on drugstore and supermarket shelves with the methapyrilene replaced by a similar agent, pyrilamine, which has not been tested for cancer activity.

The best advice for your health and sleep is to use medication rarely or not at all. Check out the possible habits or situations in your lifestyle that may rob you of sleep, or get professional help if your sleep problem is resistant to these efforts or if it is really severe.

Indigestion

About half of us will have an occasional bout of gastrointestinal distress which we may call upset stomach, gas, heartburn or indigestion. Single episodes of stomach ache are ordinarily caused by eating too much and too fast, involuntarily swallowing air, drinking too much, eating too rich, too fatty foods or eating foods such as cabbage or onions that tend to give some people gas. Food allergies, drug side effects, early pregnancy, flu or some other infection can also cause indigestion. Then there's emotional upset, such as anxiety, anger or excitement, which can put the digestive tract in turmoil.

These single and self-limiting attacks of indigestion can usually be greatly relieved by using antacids for pain and acidity, and remedies containing simethicone for excessive gas. If you get indigestion by bad eating habits or minor nervous stress, consider planning smaller meals and trying to keep your mealtime environment calm and serene. If it seems likely that the symptoms are related to mild flu or a cold, rest, eat lightly, and wait a day or two for the indigestion to go away.

If the condition doesn't clear up or you can't attribute it to any familiar cause, you should see a doctor. Danger signs include rectal bleeding or black, tarry stools; continued vomiting or throwing up blood; jaundice (yellowing of eyes and skin); extreme weakness; unexpected weight loss; sharp or shooting abdominal pains; and high fever. Any serious emotional distress that causes unrelenting digestive upset may require professional help.

Among the serious conditions that might underlie severe or recurring indigestion symptoms are ulcers; gall-bladder disease; reflux of stomach contents upward into the esophagus; liver disease; bowel obstruction or appendicitis; infections caused by salmonella or staphylococcus in the digestive tract; food poisoning; intestinal parasites such as tapeworms; inflammatory bowel disease; malabsorption (the inability of the intestines to absorb nutrients); pancreatitis; and cancer in the digestive system or other organs.

Recurring indigestion should be investigated by a doctor; simple one-time indigestion should subside in a day or so if you remove the cause; nonprescription antacids are useful for single episodes. If you have an upset stomach along with a headache, as in a hangover, it's best to avoid aspirin-containing analgesics such as fizzy pain relievers. Your already irritated stomach lining could be damaged.

Abnormal Bleeding

Any bleeding (except, of course, normal menstruation or a minor cut or wound) is abnormal and should not be neglected. Many of the causes are minor, but serious illnesses, such as hemophilia and cancer, often signal their presence through bleeding. Generalized bleeding from different sites, such as from gums, vagina, bladder and rectum, and small under-the-skin hemorrhages, call for prompt medical attention.

• Bleeding gums may signify an infection, a blood condition, vitamin C deficiency or the need to change oral-hygiene methods; in any case, you should consult your dentist. Unhealthy gums are likely to bleed in pregnancy, a time for special dental attention.

• Nosebleed, or epistaxis, may be caused by dry membranes or injury from picking at the nose. Nasal polyps (small growths) or small ruptured blood vessels also cause bleeding. Moistening salves can help prevent and treat cracked nose lining. Direct pressure (lean forward, pinch nose closed and hold until blood flow stays stopped) works for most nosebleeds; a few severe ones wind up in the doctor's office for nasal packing. Recurring nosebleeds need medical attention because nosebleed may be a signal of systemic disease.

• Blood in the urine calls for prompt medical attention. Most likely it is caused by a bladder infection that is readily treated, but serious disease such as cancer cannot be ruled out.

• Rectal bleeding, if it comes from a familiar hemorrhoid or a rectal scratch and is a single episode, may be unimportant. But bowel bleeding is a serious sign and should be taken up with your physician. Either bright-red blood or tarry black stool may indicate intestinal or rectal bleeding.

• Easy bruising, which amounts to bleeding within tissues, can point toward various vitamin deficiencies. Also, it occurs more often in older people as blood vessels become fragile. If it is not accompanied by other abnormal bleeding, it probably will not turn out to be serious; but if you continue to bruise too easily, it's a good idea to ask your physician about it.

• "Spiders," or telangiectasia, and varicose veins on the legs happen to many normal and healthy people and tend to run in families. Alcoholics and people with nutritional deficiencies are also susceptible. Support hose can help delay and relieve the aches caused by sagging leg veins. Surgical stripping may be done in severe cases. In injection treatment, the trapped blood that's causing the discoloration is pushed out and replaced by a salt solution, after which the discolored vein segment collapses and is absorbed. It can be effective as cosmetic treatment. The trouble is, additional little purple veins usually keep appearing. (See also Chapter 11.)

• Vaginal bleeding can mean different things at different times of life and in various situations. Irregular spotting can occur in young women who occasionally have a missed ovulation, or it may happen to women on low-dose oral contraceptives, or after intercourse when there's a vaginal infection, or it can be caused by a uterine polyp. Many women have some spotting early in pregnancy. If this should happen to you—if such bleeding is heavier than a normal period, or if you feel faint or discharge any tissue—get immediate medical attention. If the bleeding is light, go to bed and call your doctor. Later in pregnancy, spotting may occur after intercourse. Any bleeding at all at this time should be reported to your physician.

In women of menopausal age, any vaginal bleeding should be reported to a physician. Cyclic bleeding, however, can be expected in postmenopausal women taking replacement estrogens in an interrupted cycle.

Anxiety

We all feel anxious at times. When it's a normal and rational feeling, anxiety pushes us to perform, helps us to learn and appreciate the events of our lives. We need the sense of anxiety to distinguish what's going wrong from what's going right. But excessive anxiety can stop us in our tracks, deprive us of the ability to cope, drain the joy out of life and lead to genuine illness.How do we prevent or avoid the crippling kind of anxiety and combat it if it occurs?

Here are some preliminary steps to take in dealing with situational stress.

• Sort out the things you believe are causing stress, isolate them, identify them—all of them.
• Talk through each factor with someone who is sympathetic and close to you.

• Work out plans for dealing with each stress factor separately, a little at a time if you have to.

• In those plans, try to include some new activity, maybe even a change of scene—an absence from everyday routine can often do wonders.

• If you see no improvement, don't hesitate: seek professional counseling.

When you decide to get help, you'll want to be sure the therapist is qualified, competent and responsible. Unfortunately, in most states almost any person can set himself up in business as a "therapist" with no license or training; and obviously such persons could compound your personal problems instead of helping. Here are some steps you can take to locate a qualified therapist:

• Ask your physician for referral.

• Call your community or county Mental Health Association; ask if they have a patient referral service.

• Call your nearest medical college or large medical center. Ask the department of psychology or psychiatry to guide you to a qualified mental-health referral service.

• In the Yellow Pages, see "Mental Health Information and Treatment Centers." Follow up on those that are community- or government-affiliated.

• Call your nearest family-service agency that is accredited by the Family Service Association of America. This can generally be found in the Yellow Pages under "Marriage and Family Counselors."

• Under the same Yellow Page listing, see counseling agencies sponsored by the church of your choice.

Muscle and Bone Pain

When you hurt a muscle, the first step is to wrap the injured part in a cold compress for at least half an hour. Ice wrapped in a towel, never applied directly to skin, is an effective cold pack. If there is swelling, keep applying cold packs for several hours. When the swelling finally goes down, though the muscle will still be sore, a comforting warm—not hot—shower or soak in the tub will help take out the soreness. Two aspirin taken every four hours can reduce pain and inflammation.

When you injure a bone, the first step is to check for a possible fracture. If you can't move the injured member or it appears distorted, put a cool pack on it and start for the nearest doctor or hospital emergency room at once. When it's only a bad bruise, apply cold compresses for several hours to reduce swelling and hematoma (bleeding inside the injured tissues).

Aches and pains in the joints not caused by injuries used to be generally called rheumatism; now they're more likely to be called arthritis. Strictly speaking, arthritis means inflammation of the joints, and the term covers a wide range of different disorders. There are literally dozens of causes for arthritic pain, including gout, gonorrhea, tumors and connective-tissue diseases, to name some serious ones.

A minor temporary ache or pain in a muscle, joint or bone usually gets better fast with rest, warmth and aspirin. But if it gets worse, lasts more than a couple of days or sets off other symptoms such as fever, check in with your doctor.

An important pointer for people who have ongoing arthritic pain: there is no need to, as many do, engage in a lonely battle against advancing disability and pain. More than 37 million Americans suffer from some form of the disease (there are five major forms of arthritis, each with different causes, different treatment).

Lower-Back Pain

Pain in the lower spine is very common. It may be centered in the lumbar, lumbosacral or sacroiliac (medical terms for particular groups of vertebrae) regions of the spine. It may also shoot down the backs of the legs, along the great sciatic nerve, largest in the body. This does not necessarily mean the nerve is being pinched.

There is a lot of medical disagreement on the best treatment for lower-back pain and its related problems. Surgery, manipulation of the spine, exercises, rest and drugs, and injections all have their advocates.

Lower-back pain may come from faulty posture or may occur when the posture is excellent. It may be caused by a mechanical fault in the spine's structure, such as scoliosis (a slightly rotated spine); from overweight, lack of exercise or advancing age. In older women, pain in any part of the spinal area can result from osteoporosis, or thinning bone, which causes crush fractures and collapse of weakened vertebrae. Acute pain may come from a lower-back sprain after lifting a heavy object, twisting the body the wrong way, or just bending over.

"Slipped disk" is a serious back problem, often so acutely painful and disabling that medical assistance is a must. The disk—cartilage material that separates the bony vertebrae—can slip or squeeze out of its place when its supporting ligaments weaken. When a disk "goes out," there's nothing to do but get medical attention. The specialty field that deals with this problem is orthopedics.

Constipation

First let us discard the idea that a "daily bowel movement" is essential. The amount of stool depends entirely on the amount of indigestible material eaten; the frequency depends on the filling of the colon that brings on the urge to defecate. If you take a small amount of fiber, or bulk, in your diet, you will produce smaller and less frequent bowel movements. With a high-fiber diet you will have larger and more frequent movements. Perfectly normal bowel frequencies can vary all the way from three times a day to once in three days.

Constipation, or difficult, delayed passage of bowel movements, for most people is a temporary condition that can be managed by increasing the intake of bulk and water.

Chronic constipation happens to some older people, to people who have a laxative habit, and to people who habitually ignore the urge to defecate, so that rectal sensitivity becomes dulled and the signal no longer functions. Pregnant women often have constipation because the enlarging uterus crowds the bowel and rectum, and digestive action also is slowed by the pregnancy process. Constipation also can trigger hemorrhoids.

If you think you have constipation, add some bran to your diet in cereal or bread products. Eat lots of whole grains, fruit and vegetables. Be sure you drink generous amounts of fluids. When the urge to defecate comes, attend to it promptly. When you have a bad bout of constipation, causing cramps, an occasional laxative may be used. But regular use of laxatives can make mild constipation worse and can interfere with absorption of vitamins and other nutrients.

Diarrhea

One very sensible defense mechanism of the body is to get spoiled food through the system and out, fast. Almost all of us have had an occasional bout of diarrhea due to infected food, and it is believed that thousands of cases of mild intestinal upset are simple food poisoning. A good many factors can cause failure of the colon to do its routine job of converting the liquid contents of the gut to solids; among them, protozoal infection such as traveler's diarrhea from contaminated food or water, bacteria or viruses, antibiotic treatment, excessive use of laxatives, or an emotional crisis.

If you have only one or two loose or fluid bowel movements, and feel all right otherwise or as though you have only a minor viral illness, drink plenty of water, eat lightly and expect to feel fine in a day or so. But if the attack is so severe that you are prostrated, if the diarrhea persists for days or is extremely frequent, if there's blood or any small egglike objects in the stool, or if you have additional symptoms such as fever or headache, call your physician promptly.

Depression

Although it is no fun to feel depressed, it is not necessarily bad. A depressed period can be a useful time to think things through, or even to restructure one's life. Like anxiety, depression as a rational response helps us to see some things more clearly.

But depression that stops one from living or thinking normally, or that leads to self-destructive thoughts, is serious indeed and requires help. Many people don't recognize their symptoms as those of depression. They may go to their doctor with complaints of stomach trouble, pain, insomnia or other symptoms, but fail to say anything about their feelings of depression.

A few years back, depression was considered strictly psychological. Today scientists are convinced that a good share of depressive illness is actually biological, perhaps due to hormone shifts in the chemistry of the brain. When this is the case, drug treatment can often set the balance right.

Signs of oncoming depression that you may observe either in yourself or in someone else include loss of pleasure in things once greatly enjoyed; loss of appetite; loss of sex drive; changes in sleeping patterns; fatigue, especially in daytime. The body's energy systems are simply out of phase.

Even when depression has an organic cause it may be set off by something else, such as a disappointment, that may seem to be the actual cause. But in this state your reaction to the troubling event can be greatly exaggerated. If you think you are suffering from depression, if things look generally bleak and you have a sense of not being able to cope, do reach for help. Tell your doctor about your feelings as well as your symptoms. Get in touch with a qualified mental-health center (as discussed in the section on anxiety). Don't rely on alcohol or medications to pick up your spirits (alcohol is, in fact, a depressant). And don't feel guilty if you are depressed; your feelings are not due to something you did wrong.

Palpitations

The sense of fluttering in the chest, or the feeling of a skipped heartbeat followed by a big thump, can be frightening. Premature heartbeats, medically called extrasystoles, are one cause of erratic heart rhythm. Many of us have these occasional extra beats, and in the absence of diagnosable heart disease, extrasystoles are not dangerous at all. But where there is heart disease, premature beats are considered an added risk factor.

A bout of pitter-patters or skip-thumps may be set off by pain elsewhere in the body by emotion or fatigue, or by ingredients in coffee, tea, liquor or tobacco smoke. These incidents may become more frequent as you get older. If you have worrisome heart palpitations, see your doctor to learn whether the extra beats are associated with other coronary signs or whether you can ignore them as harmless butterflies.

Anemia

In times past when a woman was somewhat pale and inclined to be listless she was described as "anemic." The most common form of anemia, caused by iron deficiency, can result from pregnancy, from heavy menstrual loss of blood or from a poor diet. The solution, of course, is replenishment of the body's iron stores. Supplemental iron in the form of pills or capsules should be prescribed by a physician because the dosage is correlated with hemoglobin levels and geared to the blood's capacity for taking in iron. Excessive iron is harmful to the digestive tract.

Foods that supply iron in a form the body can readily absorb include fortified cereals and wheat germ, liver and lean beef. The iron in dried beans and some other plant sources is not as plentiful as in animal sources; but strangely enough, if beans and meat are eaten in the same dish or meal, almost the total amount of iron can be absorbed. In spinach, alas, the iron is locked up by oxalic acid and hardly any of it gets into your bloodstream.

Authorities agree that pregnant women need supplemental iron, since even the ideal diet cannot fill the iron demands of both mother and fetus. Even women who are not pregnant should have a test as part of their general checkup. When iron levels stay low in spite of iron supplementation, physicians look for other reasons.

Pernicious anemia, a severe disease, is less common than iron-deficiency anemia and usually occurs in older people. It is treated by injections of vitamin B_{12}. Anemia can also be caused by deficiencies of folic acid (a vitamin found in green leafy vegetables, yeast, liver and mushrooms), by deficiencies of other vitamins such as C, or of protein. Pregnant women and women taking oral contraceptives are subject to anemia due to folic acid and vitamin B_6 deficiencies. They should have either a diet high in B_6 and folate or supplements of these vitamins. Other, rarer forms of anemia are related to bone-marrow disorders and abnormalities in the production of red blood cells; they include sickle-cell disease and thalassemia (another hereditary anemia).

About Mood Drugs

Fatigue, headache, insomnia, indigestion: these and many more of
the familiar ailments may arise from direct causes such as unwise
eating or overwork. They may also be, and very often are, distress
signals of anxiety or depression. Genuine organic illness—high
blood pressure, stomach ulcers, bowel spasm, for example—can
result from emotional upset that goes on and on, often as a reaction
to some problem one cannot solve or does not want to confront.

Mood-changing drugs—tranquilizers, sedatives, antidepressants
—are being taken by the billions of doses to help people get out of
emotional discomfort. Surveys of the uses of legal, prescribed drugs
for mood relief show that women are the major users—consuming
80 percent of amphetamines (as "uppers" or weight-losing aids), 67
percent of tranquilizers, 60 percent of barbiturates.

As anybody knows who has ever taken a pill to relieve stress, the
drug cannot cure the problem that caused the stress. Lino Covi,
M.D., at Johns Hopkins Medical Center, has explained the proper
medical reasons for prescribing these drugs: "Severe anxiety and
depression should first be relieved pharmacologically, and then one
gets at the underlying causes with basic psychotherapy." Dr. Covi
pointed out that in less severe cases, 25 to 30 percent of patients can
be relieved without medication.

The risk, of course, lies in continuing to use drugs *instead* of
coping with the causes of stress. Even moderate social drinking
compounds the danger of mood drugs. When one wants to stop
using some of the mood drugs, severe to violent withdrawal symptoms can occur if the drug has been used for an extended time. It's
important to know, for example, that with tranquilizers, withdrawal
symptoms can occur several days after the last pill has been taken.
You may feel fine for a few days; then comes a bad stretch which
may seem like the old problem back again—the one for which you
started drug treatment. But these symptoms most likely will vanish
after about forty-eight hours, and when they do occur, are not
nearly as punishing as withdrawal reactions of barbiturates or nar-
cotics. And if you've been on any mood-altering medication for a
prolonged period, your physician may direct you in tapering-off the
doses—a schedule you should follow to the letter.

PART II

THE FERTILE YEARS

Most women have no characters at all.

—Alexander Pope,
Moral Essays, *Epistle II*

Although our gender is not the sole, salient fact about us, it's an important fact, and one in which to rejoice. The female reproductive system is our proud possession; it deserves our understanding and our best care. But it is not, as some antiquated authorities believed, the totality of the female person.

Nor is a woman helplessly at the mercy of her gonadal cycles and organs, a misapprehension that brought on a hilarious political flap back in 1970. Edgar Berman, M.D., a physician who sat on a party committee for deciding national priorities, stated that menstrual periods and menopause make women unfit to hold down important, decision-making jobs. Moreover, he felt, women's rights as a political issue wasn't "important enough to be brought into a serious discussion of national problems." Challenged, Dr. Berman retreated into ever deeper, hotter water by accusing a congresswoman of "raging hormonal imbalance" because she disagreed with him. Other physicians, male as well as female, deplored Dr. Berman's views. Said a prominent woman obstetrician-gynecologist, " 'Folklore' is a good word for it." (Under the pressure of fellow members, the doctor reluctantly resigned from the priorities committee.)

Belief in women's biological thralldom may not yet be entirely erased from the minds of men—or even some women; but it's being taken less and less seriously, and more and more women see clearly that gender need not stand in the way of equality.

As women began untying their aprons, they also began to destroy some health myths that had served only to reinforce their societal shackles and had often worked to the detriment of feminine health and well-being. Among the myths: that the menstrual cycle is fairly fraught with physical disability; that emotional limitations accompany the state of womanhood and are prevalent during the menses; and that pregnancy is a somewhat morbid, if inevitable and important, condition.

An example of such a health myth is built right into our language. "Hysteria"—a state characterized by excitability and loss of control —is derived from the Greek word for uterus, a word that also lingers in "hysterectomy" and "hysterotomy." Hysterical behavior was once believed to occur only in women and to be caused by an inflammation of the womb.

Another example of the attitude toward women reflected in language (this time Latin) is the medical and anatomical term "pudendum," applied to the female external genital organs, which include the labia, clitoris, pubic mound and vaginal vestibule. The term literally means "that of which one ought to be ashamed."

In this section we will focus on the reproductive organs and the way they really work. We will begin with menarche, the first menstrual period, and investigate the ongoing, cyclic nature of our human ovulatory system. We will discuss pregnancy and the health and well-being of both the mother and the unborn child. We will also explore the options in preventing and controlling pregnancy, as well as problems of infertility among people who want babies. We will examine the major disease problems of the reproductive tract —except cancer, which is covered in Chapter 14 in terms applicable to women of all ages. Finally, we will consider the minor, common symptoms and complaints that are related to the female organs and the ovulatory cycle and tell how they can best be managed or prevented.

5

THE FIRST PERIOD AND MENSTRUATION

Ask your mother about it, then ask your grandmother—virtually every woman alive can give a vivid account of the time she began to menstruate. Many stories are pitiful; the bewilderment, shame and terror that shadow the youngster's life for a long time. Other tales are funny, but only in retrospect; full of old-fashioned notions about menstruation, now largely abandoned. And still other accounts—usually those of more recent date—are endearing and amusing, about girls or a girl and her mother sharing the excitement and nervousness of the long awaited, much discussed first period.

It's called menarche (from the Greek for "month" and "beginning") and is pronounced *menARKy*. After this first instance of menstruation, or bloody discharge from the vagina, the menstrual period usually recurs with clocklike regularity every four weeks or so, but sometimes it will skip around and not come again for several months to a year or more.

A fascinating book on menstruation and menstrual customs is *The Curse*, by Emily Toth, Ph.D., Janice Delaney, Ph.D., and Mary Jane Lupton, Ph.D. During their research on this subject the authors found that even today about 20 percent of adolescent girls are uninformed about the menarche when it happens. This means that one out of every five young girls is being taken by surprise at the first menstrual bleeding, each one almost certainly convinced that something is terribly wrong with her body.

The attitude of a girl's mother and her example and ability to counsel her child on the approach of menarche are profoundly influential. If the mother is habitually disabled by her own menstrual periods, if she regards "the curse" as a burden, an illness, or as something disgusting and shameful, it's going to be difficult for her daughter to avoid the same attitude.

But not inevitably. With today's greater openness and candor about the body and about sexual behavior, and with much more information readily available in print and on film, a girl has a good chance to learn the facts about her menstrual cycle and to develop a healthy, positive attitude toward it.

An 1897 manual, *What a Young Girl Ought to Know,* quoted by author Stephen Kern in his book *Anatomy and Destiny,* throws some light on the inhibitions and prohibitions that were imposed on our mothers and grandmothers. Children were forbidden ever to discuss their bodies with each other:

"The little girl who values her modesty . . . will never allow anyone to talk to her concerning any part of her body in a way that is not sweet and pure." Instead, the girl is to tell other children: "I would rather you would not tell me about it. I will ask my mother . . . Mother tells me everything that I ought to know and she tells it to me in such a way that makes it very sweet to me, and so I have my little secrets with mother, and not with other girls."

But the very existence of this syrupy but threatening manual intended for the mother to present to her daughter, as well as many equally quaint guidebooks for married ladies, seems to indicate that mothers themselves were in no position to impart "what a young girl ought to know."

The same manual warned that masturbation would leave a mark on a girl's face that "those who are wise" could recognize, that it could also be detected by naughty behavior and unnatural appetites —for mustard, pepper, vinegar and spices—and that evil thoughts create actual poisons in the blood.

These days, girls are reaching menarche earlier than their mothers and grandmothers; and they are taller and larger for their age than the girls of earlier times. Menarche now appears when a girl is between twelve and thirteen years old. But it is perfectly normal to start menstruation as early as ten or as old as seventeen. The growing-up scenario for girls goes something like this:

- First comes a growth spurt to enable the body to reach its full height before the sex hormones begin their action and curtail the growth of the long bones.
- Next, adult female curves appear. Breasts may pop up at an amazing rate, or they may stay small and many girls worry about whether they will *ever* need a brassiere. Hips grow; if a girl is thin, her waist will become spectacularly narrow, but at the same time her buttocks may jut out.
- The breasts will almost certainly be sore and painful at times. They may seem caked and hard inside.
- Hair sprouts in the armpits and across the genital area. The legs may become hairy enough to need shaving. Oily facial skin is a problem, and pimples appear.
- Finally, the period arrives. It may be simple and easy, or it may bring some discomfort or pain. It may return right on time the next month, but for many girls it takes time to settle down to monthly regularity.

The start of the menstrual cycle is the signal that the body is capable of reproduction. Research has found that some girls who become sexually active while they are quite young may have intercourse many times without using contraception and mistakenly conclude they can't get pregnant. But as their bodies mature, the potential for pregnancy grows, and sooner or later it's very likely that there will be conception. Therefore it's always wise to think that pregnancy is a distinct possibility with unprotected intercourse.

The Menstrual Cycle

Menstrual flow is still being described in some medical school classes as "the weeping of a disappointed uterus." This poetic idea supposes that a woman's body craves a continuous state of pregnancy, which is, Lewis Carroll would say, "a sentiment open to doubt."

HORMONES

Estrogen is a "female hormone" that produces a variety of what are considered feminizing changes. Actually "estrogen" refers to an entire class of female hormones, some of which are naturally produced and some of which are synthetic. All of the estrogens have some effects in common: they stimulate the lining of the uterus in preparation for ovulation; they stimulate thickness and depth of the vaginal walls; they stimulate the breasts. In addition, they have subtle effects on almost every organ in the body; skin, hair, liver and blood all are affected by estrogens. Generally, estrogens are made in the ovaries, although they can also be made in the skin or fatty tissues.

Progestin is a female hormone which is produced by the ovary (or the placenta during pregnancy). **_Progesterone_** is one type of progestin. Progestins stimulate the lining of the uterus and prepare the body in a variety of subtle ways for a pregnancy.

Oral contraceptives contain both estrogens and progestins, mimicking to some extent the hormones normally produced in a female. The ups and downs of estrogens during an ordinary menstrual cycle account for many of the symptoms women have with their periods, such as weight gain due to water retention, headaches and nausea.

Androgens are male hormones. All women have some male hormones; however, if these hormones become excessive, deepening of the voice, abnormal hair growth, and acne may result.

Let us trace the cycle from its start at the base of the brain. There the pituitary gland, order-giver of the body, sends a follicle-stimulating hormone (FSH) into the bloodstream.* When FSH reaches the ovaries it seems to select a single follicle, or egg capsule, which starts to grow. Meanwhile the pituitary has sent along another hormone, luteinizing hormone (LH), which works along with FSH to produce estrogens, such as estradiol, inside the follicle and hurry along

*The pituitary is actually responding to messages from the hypothalamus (part of the midbrain) and higher brain centers mediated through LH and FSH or gonadotropin releasing hormones (LHRH, FSHRH or GRH).

its development. At the same time the lining of the uterus is thickening into a plushy pocket, rich in blood vessels, designed to be a proper nesting site for any fertilized egg that may come along.

The pituitary now orders a decrease in FSH and increased LH. About fourteen days after the beginning of the cycle the follicle ruptures, the mature egg is pushed out of the ovary and picked up by the nearby Fallopian tube. The follicle that has just been left now transforms itself into an actual organ, called the corpus luteum, or yellow body. It gets busy making still another hormone, progesterone. This hormone works on the uterine lining still further, getting it ready for the expected egg. The entire system is waiting for a sperm to fertilize the precious egg during its promenade down the tube.

But—since we're describing the menstrual period—fertilization

HORMONAL CHANGES OF THE MENSTRUAL CYCLE

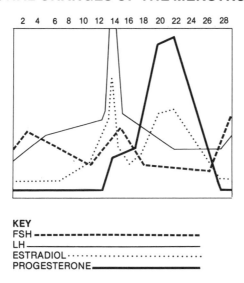

KEY
FSH ----------------------------
LH ————————————
ESTRADIOL ·
PROGESTERONE ————————

About day 13, estrogen rises, triggering the "LH surge." Ovulation occurs usually within twenty-four hours. Progesterone and estrogen levels build up; uterine lining thickens. Nine to eleven days later, sharp drop in estrogen and progesterone causes uterine lining to collapse, bringing on menstrual flow.

Based on The CIBA Collection of Medical Illustrations by
Frank H. Netter, M.D. Reprinted with permission

does not happen. The corpus luteum breaks down. The lining of the uterus stops growing and is loosened and shed. The uterus discards the now superfluous cells, along with some disposable blood, into the vagina. This blood amounts to only half to three quarters of the menstrual fluid. Bits of membrane, mucus and worn-out cells make up the rest. The fluid has a great deal more calcium than regular blood, and you'll notice it doesn't clot easily. Normally you lose only a few spoonfuls of blood in a three- to five-day period. Because of its color it may seem like a great deal more. If you think you actually are bleeding excessively, talk to your physician, who can check for any unusual problems and may look for signs of iron-loss anemia and prescribe medication for you if it's needed.

What would have happened if the egg had met a sperm in the tube? The corpus luteum would have gone on working for about three months. The fertilized egg would have grabbed its spot in the rich uterine lining, and begun to grow. As soon as that wonderful

ENDOMETRIUM DURING THE MENSTRUAL CYCLE

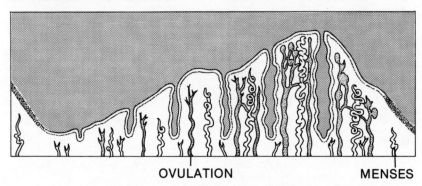

OVULATION   MENSES

Build-up of the endometrium during the menstrual cycle.

After menstruation, the endometrial lining of the uterus builds up under the influence of estrogen. The endometrial glands become long, and the blood supply becomes rich and abundant. After ovulation, the endometrium becomes even richer, with thick spiraled arteries ready to nourish the egg should it implant. During the time after ovulation, both progesterone and estrogen stimulate and maintain the endometrium. If the egg is not fertilized, estrogen and progesterone production falls sharply. The endometrium literally collapses. Blood vessels break open, and menstrual flow results. Toward the end of menses, estrogen production begins again, and the cycle starts over.

Adapted from an original painting by Frank H. Netter, M.D.,
from The CIBA Collection of Medical Illustrations, copyright by
CIBA Pharmaceutical Company, Division of CIBA-GEIGY Corporation

temporary organ, the placenta, had grown big enough, the corpus luteum would hand over to it the job of producing progesterone and would contentedly wither away.

Menstruation has been called the "friendly monthly nuisance"— as well as a lot of other things. Probably no biological event has produced so much folklore, mostly morbid, so many misguided "health" regulations or so many crude jokes. Social scientists have gathered sheaves of reports about beliefs and customs related to menstruation, in our own and in other cultures. When writing their book, *The Curse*, authors Toth, Delaney and Lupton found that menstrual taboos and hangups are still quite prevalent today; in fact, several publishers refused the book because they thought the subject was disgusting, and book reviewers criticized the authors for writing at all on the topic. Men, probably because it doesn't happen to them, have a lot of outdated views and superstitions about menstruation, the authors find. Even modern, educated men may think of a woman as "unwell" when she's menstruating.

Primitive people still observe all kinds of customs regarding menstruation, including that of isolating menstruating women in separate huts. Contamination by, or even the presence of, menstrual blood is still widely feared. It's supposed to cause crops to fail, hunting to be sparse, milk to sour, bread and cakes to fall. But the authors of *The Curse* found one culture that was different: the Navajo Indians hold a special party for each girl to celebrate her first period, with dancing and singing on the joy of becoming a woman. And the authors suggest that women might follow the Navajo example when daughters reach menarche, by making it a joyous occasion, not an anxiety-producing event.

Signs, Symptoms and Management of the Menstrual Cycle

As mentioned earlier, menstruation may bring on skin disturbances. If you're inclined to get acne, it probably will flare up when you have your period. Some women get pronounced dark circles under the eyes. Some vaginal infections get worse or are triggered by the period, most likely because the vaginal environment is less acidic then.

Ovulation, the key event that results in menstruation about two weeks later when no conception takes place, is a keenly felt stage of the cycle for some women but is not even noticed by others. Research has shown that plenty of physical events occur during the ovulatory phase. Some women experience *Mittelschmerz,* distinct abdominal pains similar to menstrual cramps. Breasts may enlarge and become tender or sore, ankles may swell, and transitory weight gains can amount to several pounds. The extra weight is actually water retained by the body.

For most women the excess fluid is disposed of naturally after a few hours' rest. For those whose fluid retentions are unusually troublesome, a doctor may prescribe a mild diuretic pill to take at this time of month. It's not a good idea to take diuretics frequently on your own; they work by causing sodium to be excreted in the urine, taking excess water with it, but they also cause the body to drop potassium, and excessive loss of this mineral can make you feel weak. Extreme depletion of potassium could be serious.

There are several useful drugs for preventing or controlling really disabling premenstrual tension (PMT). These are aimed at correcting any of a number of hormone imbalances that set off the symptoms. Women who suffer from severe PMT have been found to have unusually high levels of the hormone prolactin.

On the other hand, the mid-month ovulatory period can set off certain "highs." Careful studies show that women feel pain less and that sight, hearing and the sense of smell actually heighten. Many women have a surge of sexual excitement in connection either with ovulation or the menstrual period. Others report bursts of creative energy and increased physical well-being, or a sense of power.

Women are said to be nervous and jumpy at certain times of the menstrual cycle. It is possible that one woman's "nerves" can be another woman's "high." By recognizing the raised tension connected with the menstrual cycle, it is possible for us to use it positively instead of considering it a handicap. "The stars dispose; they do not compel," say astrology buffs. We might say the same of the influence of the moon.

Disposing of the menstrual fluid is a matter involving hygiene and comfort. Through the ages, Dr. Toth tells us, women have always used some means for taking up and disposing of menstrual blood.

Matrons of the Roman Empire used cloth bandages; primitive African and Australian women use grass or vegetable-fiber bandages. In Europe and America, before commercial sanitary napkins, absorbent "rags" were used, washed and used again. (1920, incidentally, was a great year for women in the United States. We got the vote; and we also got the first disposable sanitary pads.)

Tampons go back to ancient times, too, we're told in *The Curse*. Japanese women used paper tampons, Indonesian women made tampons from vegetable fibers, Romans had woolen tampons, and Egyptians, as you might expect, had them made of papyrus.

Young girls often believe they can't use tampons because their vaginal opening isn't large enough or that they'll lose their virginity by putting in a tampon. But one's virginity is not defined by the presence of the hymen; one is a virgin until coitus, or sexual intercourse, takes place. The hymen is simply a tissue between the developing internal and external genital organs; the "hymenal ring" has an opening of varying sizes which usually is large enough to admit a tampon. (A small number of young women have a condition called imperforate hymen in which the hymenal ring is closed and menstrual blood cannot get out. This is readily corrected in a simple surgical procedure that may be performed in a gynecologist's office.)

Today more and more young women use tampons from the start of menstruation. Some gynecologists recommend starting with tampons, for neatness, freedom from odor and to avoid the risk of irritating the exterior genital region with a napkin or pad. Yet the choice of menstrual products is wide, and each woman must decide for herself, in terms of what makes her comfortable and is most convenient. Many women use both tampons and napkins, for different times and different rates of menstrual flow. Major manufacturers offer starter kits, with a variety of their feminine products and instructions.

Using a tampon for the first time may require a fair amount of dexterity and possibly a bit of lubrication on the tip. There's no reason to fear that the tampon might accidentally enter the urinary canal—that opening is far too small. Main pointers for beginners are: Find the proper angle for inserting the tampon, neither straight upward nor straight back from the vaginal opening. A good rule is to aim toward the small of your back. Be sure the tampon is placed high enough, beyond the entrance muscles; then it will neither fall out nor give you any sensation that you're wearing it. Recently much concern has surrounded the possibility of an illness called "toxic shock syndrome," which may occur in tampon users (as well as other women and men). This is discussed in Chapter 11. In reality, millions of women have used billions of tampons with apparent safety, but tampon users should be familiar with this entity and the symptoms that are described in tampon package inserts.

Dysmenorrhea

This is the medical term for painful, difficult menstruation. Most of us experience it simply as menstrual cramps, even though it may also involve other kinds of pain, such as backache and nausea. There are two types of dysmenorrhea and they need to be understood because their causes and treatment are different. *Primary dysmenorrhea* is the kind that starts about the time of menarche, or first menstruation. *Secondary dysmenorrhea* occurs later and has either an organic or an exterior cause.

Only a few years ago, doctors and the general public believed that primary dysmenorrhea was largely psychosomatic, having a mental or emotional cause. The woman with menstrual cramps was somehow blamed for her problem. "Female weakness" was the common term. It was also believed that bad posture, physical sluggishness and neurotic attitudes toward one's femininity were causes of cramps. A medical textbook still in use states: "Functional dysmenorrhea is generally a symptom of a personality disorder, even though hormonal imbalance may be present."

Not so, says James R. Dingfelder, M.D., associate professor of obstetrics and gynecology at the University of North Carolina Medical School: "Dysmenorrhea from psychiatric causes is indeed rare in clinical practice. There's no doubt that recurring pain can affect one's attitude toward menstruation. This does not mean the attitude causes the pain, but quite the contrary."

Neither do menstrual cramps indicate there's anything wrong with your cycle. "Practically without exception," said Dr. Dingfelder. "It takes a perfectly normal menstrual cycle to grow enough endometrial lining to produce painful menstruation."

In menstrual cramping the uterus contracts too fast and too hard. This constricts the blood circulation in the uterine tissue and produces pain, as it would in any overworked muscle. Doctors now believe the uterine muscle works too hard because of overstimulation by prostaglandin, a potent hormone substance secreted by the uterine lining. Drugs that succeed in relieving menstrual pain are nearly always those that inhibit the body's production of prostaglandin. They include indomethacin, ibuprofen and other prescription drugs. Aspirin, which may help relieve cramps, is a weak prostaglandin inhibitor.

Some of the old-time remedies for cramps are effective and may help you avoid taking stronger medication. Bed rest, moist heat on the abdomen or a heating pad, and taking hot drinks are some of the old and sworn-by remedies. Exercises can be useful. Mild pain-relieving medicines are sometimes enough to relieve cramps.

The grandmotherly assurance that your menstrual cramps will abate once you have your first baby is generally true in primary dysmenorrhea. And oral contraceptives nearly always stop or greatly reduce the monthly cramps. These days, however, physicians hesitate to put a young girl on the pill purely to prevent cramps, mainly because of increased risks of circulatory problems and because it could mean many years of exposure to added estrogens.

Secondary dysmenorrhea is quite a different matter. Any menstrual pain that happens unexpectedly and well after the first menstruation should be medically investigated. Endometriosis is a condition that can cause severe cramping and sometimes causes fertility problems. In this disease, tissue similar to the endometrium, or uterine lining, grows on the surfaces of other organs such as the ovaries, Fallopian tubes and intestines, and in the vagina. These islands or implants of tissue behave like the endometrium—they thicken and break down each month in response to the hormone cycles. But because the tissues can't be neatly shed and disposed of as menstruation, the body responds by trying to absorb the excess blood. The out-of-place tissue can produce inflammation, scarring, cysts and adhesions, and can permanently damage the affected organs.

Menstrual Problems—Too Much Flow or Too Little

Aside from painful menstruation, menstrual-flow problems can be divided into two major types—too much or too little. But there are several medical terms your doctor would use to describe the different degrees and conditions of these problems. We'll define these terms, discuss the major causes of the disorders, the medical tests that are often made to determine the causative conditions, and some medical approaches aimed at putting the menstrual cycle in order.

TOO LITTLE BLEEDING: AMENORRHEA AND OLIGOMENORRHEA

Amenorrhea is the absence of menstrual flow; oligomenorrhea is scanty flow or infrequent periods. Both conditions may originate in the central nervous system and involve part of the endocrine system (the hypothalamus and the pituitary gland) or may be caused by the ovaries or the uterus. In some cases the pituitary and hypothalamus glands are the primary cause of amenorrhea, either as a result of birth defects, injury, radiation damage or tumors. Medications, particularly those for seizures or for nervous or mental disorders, can also cause amenorrhea, as can some "street drugs," such as stimulants, sedatives and tranquilizers.

Stress-induced amenorrhea can result from severe emotional pressure. Changes in environment such as moving, going away to school, or family or personal difficulties can cause the problem. When the emotional stress is relieved, periods may resume without any treatment being necessary—except perhaps the reassurance of a physician. Severe medical illness can also produce stress sufficient to cause amenorrhea.

Dietary amenorrhea is related to the physical stress of losing as much as 30 percent of body fat, 15 percent of body weight, or a loss of twenty pounds or more. In these conditions, women may stop menstruating temporarily. Underweight women often become chronically amenorrheic. Weight reduction below a certain critical body weight is believed to suppress the hypothalamic and pituitary hormones that are essential to the menstrual cycle.

Amenorrhea induced by exercise reflects a different kind of physical stress. Women in rigorous athletic training for distance running, competitive rowing and other exhausting action—not women getting moderate regular exercise—may stop menstruating.

It's likely that amenorrhea under stress had an important survival value in the evolution of mankind. When primitive tribes were in flight, or at war, or starving, they simply could not afford to have their women pregnant and bringing helpless little beings into the world. Nature may have protected those tribes by making their women temporarily infertile in stressful circumstances.

Fortunately, most amenorrhea caused by stress is temporary and readily reversed. Reducing or escaping the stress factors, gaining weight or bringing an overdemanding training schedule into moderate range usually results in spontaneous resumption of the periods. Sometimes the weight loss may be caused by a psychiatric problem, anorexia nervosa, in which an otherwise healthy young girl develops a pathologic fear of food and fat. She may lose weight until she literally starves to death. Anorexia nervosa usually requires psychiatric therapy for correcting both the weight loss and the menstrual disorder.

Extremely overweight women often become oligomenorrhic or amenorrheic. Hypothalamic and pituitary suppression may also underlie this condition, possibly as a result of the high androgen (male hormone) levels some obese women have. Except for a few women with abnormal growth of hormone-secreting tissues, in the vast majority of obese women these excess androgens (and accompanying hair growth) are the result of obesity, and not the cause.

Thyroid disorders—either high hormone output or low—can cause amenorrhea through complex hormone interactions. This is the reason that medical evaluation of menstrual problems often includes thyroid examination and testing, and when required, treatment.

When the cause of missing or scanty menstrual flow lies in the ovaries, it may be from a birth defect or from a disorder in ovarian function. It's not unusual for ovaries to simply stop releasing mature eggs before a woman reaches thirty-five, a condition called premature menopause. When ovaries must be removed surgically, the menstrual periods will of course cease; this is called surgical menopause. When ovaries or adrenal glands produce too much androgen, or male hormones, absence of flow or scanty bleeding may result, as well as excessive hairiness and other masculinizing symptoms. In these cases, hormone treatment is often indicated. In rare cases where there is a tumor, surgery may be required.

When the uterus is the source of amenorrhea, it's likely to be from cervical stenosis (narrowing of the cervical opening) or from scar tissue in the uterus. When the cervix is blocked, it is usually after an abortion, a dilation and curettage (D&C) operation, cone biopsy or cervical cauterizing. Then surgical correction is in order. The same is true where scar tissue is present or when adhesions prevent the normal build-up of endometrium. Scarring and adhesions may result from an abortion or a D&C.

If a girl has not menstruated by the time she is seventeen, her condition is described medically as primary amenorrhea. Her physician will of course investigate all possible causes, including stress and ovarian and uterine disorders. In addition, birth defects such as structural problems and genetic causes are explored.

Secondary amenorrhea, like secondary dysmenorrhea, occurs in women who have previously had normal periods.

Oral contraceptives stop menstrual bleeding in a few women. In these cases the amount of estrogen in the low-dose pills doesn't permit the endometrial lining to build up sufficiently to slough off at the end of the cycle.

Going off the pill can cause menstrual bleeding to cease, but most women restart their normal periods within a month or two after oral contraceptives are stopped. About 98 percent menstruate normally within six months. In a small number, however, amenorrhea is prolonged. Generally, it eventually returns, but some women who want to become pregnant may have to have ovulation induced with various medications.

Amenorrhea, along with breast secretion (galactorrhea), needs medical evaluation, since it could signal a tumor of the pituitary, the important endocrine gland under the middle of the brain. Most prolactin-producing pituitary tumors grow slowly and are curable, but they should be treated as early as possible.

TOO MUCH BLEEDING—DYSFUNCTIONAL UTERINE BLEEDING (DUB)
Medical descriptions of excessive menstrual flow include menorrhagia (heavy periods), metrorrhagia (bleeding between periods)

and menometrorrhagia (both conditions). Most DUB is estrogen-related, due to excessive estrogen build-up of the uterine lining or to estrogen stimulation in a noncyclic pattern. The reasons these things happen may lurk in the hypothalamus, the pituitary or the ovary, or they can be a result of medication. Some tumors secrete excess estrogen. Too much estrogen can also cause the endometrial lining to develop hyperplasia, a precancerous condition.

Excessive or unexplained bleeding can result from vaginitis (vaginal inflammation), usually as spotting after intercourse or douching. (See Chapter 9 for details on vaginitis.) Benign tumors and polyps, which are also usually benign, can cause bleeding, as can damage from a D&C, suction curettage or sterilization. Excessive bleeding that lasts for more than a few days, or that follows a D&C or a suction curettage, or that is accompanied by pain or fever, very definitely should be seen by a physician.

Until recently the D&C procedure was almost routinely used as a treatment for excessive bleeding. Stripping the uterine lining can relieve the constant shedding that accounts for some bleeding, and it may also remove any bleeding polyps that might be present. Today many physicians treat DUB with hormones, reserving surgery as a secondary treatment for younger women who are less likely than older ones to have any serious disease.

In rare instances a hysterectomy is necessary to stop severe hemorrhage. Some women, in fact, choose hysterectomy to avoid worry about bleeding episodes. Women should realize, however, that several other methods for treating DUB are available and can be tried before resorting to major surgery.

Additional Bleeding Problems

Some women who use oral contraceptives have "spotting" throughout the cycle. The doctor may handle this problem either by changing the estrogen or the estrogen/progestogen levels or by giving extra hormones during the cycle. If you have spotting, do not stop taking the pill; stay on your present pill cycle and make an appointment to see your physician. If you miss two or three pills and start to bleed, this is a perfectly normal response to cutting off estrogen. Stop your pill cycle, start using an alternate contraceptive such as

foam and condoms, and start a *new* pill pack after your bleeding
stops, or within a few days. Use the alternate contraceptive method
in addition to the pill for the next month.

Increased bleeding or cramps are fairly common complaints of
women using an intrauterine device. If there is also severe pain,
tenderness or fever, there's a possibility of infection, and you should
have the IUD removed promptly. In the absence of such trouble
signals, or of anemia, many women choose to live with the heavier
flow because they like the convenience of the IUD.

After tubal sterilization surgery, roughly 15 percent of the patients
report heavy, sometimes irregular, flow. One of the reasons may be
that these women are in the near-menopause age group, but other
causes may also exist. Diagnosis and treatment are the same as for
any other form of DUB.

Women in their late thirties and forties often have heavy or
irregular bleeding. The gradual cessation of cycling is part of the
natural process of aging in the ovary. When estrogen output is high
while cycling is diminishing, the result may be DUB. In women of
this age group, a D&C or a very careful sampling of endometrial
cells is essential to rule out the possibility of cancer. Most irregular
bleeding at this period of life is not due to any malignancy, but it
is important to check each time such irregularities occur.

Vaginitis is the usual cause of bleeding following sexual intercourse, either from vaginal infection or, in older women, from
atrophic vaginitis due to estrogen deficiency. Either form is usually
easily treated with medications inserted into the vagina, sometimes
in conjunction with antibiotics or other oral medications. But it is
important to get a medical examination for postcoital bleeding,
because it can also be a symptom of cancer in the vagina or cervix.
(See Chapter 14 for more about this.)

Vaginal bleeding in children is abnormal. It may be caused by
infection, more often by a foreign object, or by an injury from a fall
or from a sharp object. Tragically, child abuse and rape, which can
cause bleeding, are not unknown even in very small children. When
a little girl has vaginal bleeding she must have a pelvic examination
by a doctor. Because this could be both emotionally upsetting and
uncomfortable, it may be done under light anesthesia. Doctors must
report cases of child abuse to the proper authorities. In a happier

vein, it is worth noting that a newborn girl will sometimes show a small amount of vaginal bleeding. This is merely a response to extra estrogen received from her mother before birth. It will clear up without treatment.

Irregular bleeding is fairly common in newly menstruating girls. It is generally a perfectly normal event of not yet mature cyclic function, and either no treatment or a little hormone manipulation is all that's required. At one time birth-control pills were commonly prescribed to regulate periods, but this is customarily not done today, unless, of course, the girl needs contraception or the irregular flow is emotionally or physically wearing. On rare occasions, bleeding in adolescence is caused by a tumor of the ovary or central nervous system.

Sometimes rectal or urinary bleeding is confused with vaginal bleeding. To be on the safe side, any episode of this type of bleeding should be investigated by a physician. Rectal bleeding can be caused by irritation or hemorrhoids, or it may be a sign of cancer. Blood in the urine may be caused by infection or kidney stones, or it could indicate the presence of cancer.

Most women experience a menstrual disorder at some time in their lives. While irregularities can be symptoms of serious disease, the vast majority result from a slight imbalance in the finely tuned system that creates a normal menstrual flow. The female reproductive system is so elegantly designed that a small disturbance can interfere with the cycle. Considering the many possible, often trivial, causes of "too little" or "too much," the regular, normal period seems a near-miraculous event.

6

PREGNANCY AND CHILDBIRTH

A woman, after conception, during the time of her being pregnant, ought to be looked upon as indisposed or sick, though in good health: For child-bearing is a kind of nine-months' sickness.

—*From* The Master-Piece *(a manual widely sold house-to-house in the 1800s; in many homes the only guide to marriage and childbirth)*

Today, in more and more cases, the well woman is pregnant when and if she chooses to be. And she is more likely to consider her pregnant state a normal and healthy one, and the impending delivery a natural event.

But far from ignoring or neglecting her pregnancy, she wants available to her the benefits of health counseling, the watchfulness of medical examinations throughout pregnancy, and the advantages of medical technology, such as amniocentesis, when special needs arise.

The decade of the 1970s brought a veritable upheaval in the customary ways of conducting a pregnancy and delivering a child. In the 1960s, many physicians dictated the rate of weight gain the pregnant patient was permitted (usually very low) to ensure an easier delivery and supposedly to avert dangerous complications. Today, the approach has changed. We know that severe weight restriction in pregnancy leads to low-weight babies and related risks to them, as well as nutritional deficiencies for both mother and child.

A generation back, drugs for pregnancy symptoms were freely prescribed, and nonprescription remedies were also freely taken.

Today, except in special conditions, physicians restrict the use of sedatives, stimulants, tranquilizers, digestive aids and even aspirin during the various stages of pregnancy.

Finally, the prevailing styles of childbirth are undergoing drastic changes, away from the heavily drugged, routinized hospital procedure and toward more participation by both mother and father in the birth process, and "rooming in" of baby with mother during the hospital stay.

Currently there is much medical controversy, confusion and plain uproar about conditions surrounding childbirth. Rebelling against overmedicated, institutionalized, depersonalized conditions for delivery, some women have decided to forgo formal medical care and simply have their babies at home, with or without trained assistance. In some medical circles the home-birth trend is viewed with alarm, and predictions are made that there will be sharp rises in sickness and death among both mothers and babies. Between these two positions, positive developments are occurring: advances are being made not just in the health and safety of childbirth but in providing the conditions for a happy, emotionally secure start for the new parent-baby relationship. Having a baby today is more fun, more rewarding and safer than it was even a decade ago.

Before Pregnancy*

You're planning to become pregnant. If you've been on oral contraceptives, you'll naturally discontinue using them. Gynecologic authorities urge a waiting period of two to three months before you allow yourself to conceive, meanwhile using a barrier contraceptive such as the diaphragm or having your husband use a condom. The reason for this pill-free interlude is to allow the pill-induced hormonal effects on the genital organs to dissipate, thereby lowering the risks of abnormalities in the fetus. According to some research, there are also metabolic reasons for having oral contraceptives well out of your system before launching the pregnancy; the pill can cause a functional shortage of some vitamins, such as folates, B_6 and pyridoxine, and it is a good idea to be in excellent physical condition

*See Chapter 8 for information concerning conception and increasing your chances of conceiving.

nutritionally when you start a pregnancy. While trying to conceive, avoid *all* medications not medically necessary. Consult your physician about any drugs you take *before* trying to conceive.

When You Think You're Pregnant

Whether you're trying to become pregnant, trying not to, or are shuffling about somewhere in between—it's important to be alert for a missed or late period. Here, a long-term habit of marking your personal calendar on the first day of menstruation each month is an incomparable aid. If your cycles are irregular, you learn the approximate range of variation; if you're like clockwork, you'll know precisely when your next period should occur.

When it seems clear that your period is overdue, you'll want to find out if pregnancy is really the cause, by choosing (1) to see your doctor or (2) to use one of the home-test kits for pregnancy that you can buy in a drugstore.

Home kits usually consist of materials for a one- or two-hour urine test, with detailed instructions on how to do it. A few drops of early-morning urine are added to a tube containing chemical agents, along with a measured amount of purified water. You shake the tube for a specific length of time, place it on its stand and leave it undisturbed for a precise period of time. If you are pregnant, a dark-brown ring appears at the bottom of the tube. A cloudy or unspecified result is assumed to be negative.

Urine tests measure the presence of a hormone, HCG, that increases sharply very early in pregnancy. The tests are designed to detect pregnancy two weeks after a missed period. If you follow directions exactly, the test should be close to 97 percent accurate in cases of positive readings. If the reading is negative, you're only 80 percent certain of no pregnancy, so if a menstrual period doesn't start, a second test is recommended a week later. If that test is negative and you still have no period, it is urgent that you see a physician: an ectopic, or tubal pregnancy (a pregnancy outside the uterus, usually in a Fallopian tube) will not register in the home test, and if you have one, you need immediate medical care.

If you go directly to your physician for an examination instead of using a home test, he will probably give you a similar urine test or a blood test (accurate at the time of a missed period), plus a physical examination and advice. Your doctor can tell a lot about the possibility of pregnancy from observing physical signs, such as changes in your breasts and uterus.

Using a home test can be a boon if you want an instant answer as to whether or not you're pregnant and you can't get a doctor's appointment that soon. But seeing your doctor gives you the advantages of getting a physical checkup and the skilled observation of a physician. Whichever you choose, and if you are planning on having the baby, it is important to begin prenatal care at the earliest possible moment.

Pregnancy Symptoms

> *If a little feeling of pain doth runne up and downe the lower belly and about the navell, if shee be sleepy, if she loath the embracings of a man, and if her face bee pale, it is a token that she hath conceived.*
>
> —Collected Works, *Ambroise Paré*
> *(1510–1590), printed in English 1634*

You would be unusual if you got very far into pregnancy without symptoms. About four out of five pregnant women have some nausea, or "morning sickness," at some time. These transient upsets are attributed to a kind of hunger and are usually relieved by eating. You're most likely to wake up with a case of pregnancy wobblies. A couple of crackers or some dry Melba toast placed at your bedside the night before can be a real comfort in the morning. A cheerful fact about morning sickness: by the third month it has almost always passed.

The Start of Life: One Cell to Millions

From earliest times and in every culture, people have been fascinated by the marvelous process that is the making of a baby. Biology, medicine, religion and law have all probed the origins of human life. In one of the books of his *Collected Works,* entitled *Of the Generation of Man,* the French surgeon Ambroise Paré described the early embryo as an assemblage of three bubbles, which soon become the liver, heart and brain. The greater portion of the "seede," or fertilized ovum, goes into the brain, Paré believed, because this is clearly the most important part, "seate of the senses, and mansion of the minde and reason." Not until all the members of the fetus are perfectly formed does the soul or mind enter the body, Paré wrote; and he believed this happened about the fortieth day in male children, and about the forty-fifth in females. (Though no evidence backed it, it was important for the establishment of that time to believe that male babies developed faster and were stronger than females.)

In the four centuries that followed, we have learned a great deal more about the growth of the human fetus.

The human ovum—the mature egg a woman produces more or less regularly once in each of some 360 months between menarche and menopause—is the largest single cell of the human body. It ranges between a tenth to a fifth of a millimeter across (one millimeter is about the diameter of a paper-clip wire).

The human spermatozoon, on the other hand, is the body's smallest cell, but hundreds of millions of them are produced to compete for a single egg. Only one of them—a tiny, whip-tailed tadpole of a creature—wins the intrauterine race upward through the Fallopian tubes against its brothers, penetrates the ready egg and sets off the beginning of a new life.

What happens to the millions of wiggling suitors who lose the race? All of them die very shortly, of course. Many have raced mistakenly up the wrong Fallopian tube—the side where the egg wasn't, at least not this month. Bad luck. Of the sperm cells that did race toward the egg, those just behind the winner bump into something tough, for the instant the winning sperm cell enters, the ovum magically surrounds itself with a "fertilization membrane" that acts as a barrier against the also-rans.

After the meeting of egg and sperm, the fertilized ovum begins the process of cell division, splitting in two, then four, and so on, each new cell having its own specific destiny. While this is occurring the ovum is moving purposefully down the Fallopian tube to attach itself, in a week or so, to the wall of the uterus. At this point you probably still haven't a clue that you're pregnant.

The tiny embryo's way toward becoming a baby continues in the following manner:

THIRD WEEK
Beginning of brain and spinal cord appear inside the egg sac, as dividing cells start to differentiate into specific tissues.

FOURTH WEEK
Two buds punch their way outward on either side of the embryo. They will become arms. A tiny flickering in the middle marks the already beating heart. The circulation and digestive systems are beginning to form. Segments of spine are quite recognizable. The embryo is now about one fifth of an inch long.

DEVELOPMENT OF FETUS

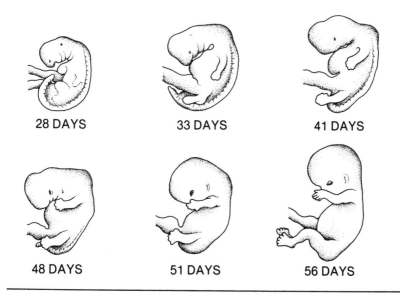

| 28 DAYS | 33 DAYS | 41 DAYS |

| 48 DAYS | 51 DAYS | 56 DAYS |

Rapid growth and development of the fetus take place during the first trimester of your pregnancy. The circulation and digestive systems begin to form. During the fifth week, arms with hands and fingers take shape, as do legs with feet and toes. By the seventh week the fetus has a face: eyes, nose, lips and tongue. At the end of the third month the fetus is over three inches long and weighs about an ounce.

FIFTH WEEK

The brain has divisions. Arms with small hands and fingers are taking shape, as are legs with feet and toes. Big dark eyes appear. The body still has quite a long tail. It measures two fifths of an inch —double its length the week before.

SIXTH WEEK

The heart now beats fast and strongly. The liver shows up in its proper place, ready to work. Little ears have sprouted. The fetal blood circulates independently of the mother's.

SEVENTH WEEK

The fetus now has its very own face, with eyes, nose, lips, tongue. Tooth buds are forming in the jaw tissues. Muscles and delicate skin have evolved. Bones are forming inside the small, perfect hands. The body is one inch long and definitely looks like a baby.

EIGHTH WEEK

There are eyelids now. Soon they'll close and remain so until the seventh month. The fetus weighs less than one tenth of an ounce —the same as three paper clips. Now you may begin to feel some standard pregnancy symptoms.

THIRD MONTH

The fetus is over three inches long, weighs a whole ounce. Its ears, eyelids, fingers and toes are fully developed and will grow from now on. The wee one swims freely at the end of its umbilical lifeline, exercising, resting, possibly practicing games it will play later, outside.

FOURTH MONTH

The little bud of a genital organ now becomes a penis or a clitoris, with a suitable scrotum or labia. But the question "Which?" was decided ages before, at the instant the sperm and egg met. At four months the unborn one is about six inches long, weighs perhaps seven ounces, is busy with hands and feet; pawing, kicking, exploring the inner surface of its world. Over much of its body the baby is covered by downy fur called lanugo. The fur will fall out before the end of the term, though some premature babies wear their dark fuzzy coats into the outside world, astonishing their parents and other relatives.

In Training: Things to Avoid

Nine calendar months. Ten lunar months. Thirty-nine weeks. Beginning at the earliest possible moment—or even better, before you become pregnant—there are useful and rewarding ground rules for taking care of yourself and your baby.

Don't smoke. Recent research indicates that cigarette smoking during pregnancy is a lot more harmful to the fetus than was formerly believed. Nicotine, the addictive drug in tobacco, may constrict the blood vessels supplying the uterus, reducing the amount of oxygen the fetus gets. In the blood itself, carbon monoxide can build up, reducing the oxygen supply still more.

Statistically, smoking mothers produce lower-weight babies, and infants born weighing less than they should are at a great disadvantage. The infant death rate is 27 percent higher in babies born to smokers than to nonsmokers. Your risk of complications is greatly increased if you smoke. The risk of miscarriage almost doubles. If you are a smoker and fear you can't break the habit, consider a smoking-cessation clinic.

Don't drink. Very high rates of physical deformity and mental retardation have been recorded in babies born to heavy-drinking mothers. But in fine-line research covering the whole range of drinking behavior, alcoholism investigators expected to find that a little wine or a single cocktail would be perfectly all right for pregnant women. Not so. The risk of the full-blown fetal alcohol syndrome, with its severe birth defects, begins with intakes of about three ounces of alcohol—half a dozen drinks a day. But incidence of parts of the syndrome, including deformities, growth problems and brain damage, can occur on as little as two drinks daily. Alcohol is a drug that crosses the placenta and readily goes into the fetal bloodstream. Official advice from the National Institute on Alcohol Abuse and Alcoholism is for women to shun alcohol entirely throughout pregnancy. Those who insist on drinking are beseeched not to have more than two drinks in any one day, and to avoid weekend drinking. If you intend to become pregnant, it's best to stop drinking before you try to conceive. You may not know you're pregnant for two weeks or more, during the critical early-development stages of the fetus, when even a slight exposure to alcohol could be damaging.

Don't smoke pot. The evidence against marijuana smoking in pregnancy is not as strong as that against tobacco, but experiments with animals, and the knowledge that the active agent of marijuana, tetrahydrocannabinol (THC), has definite effects on cell proteins and on the placenta, would indicate caution.

Stay away from your medicine chest. In the 1960s the world learned by tragic experience the effects on unborn young of the drug thalidomide, widely used in Europe and thought a harmless and helpful tranquilizer for jumpy, upset pregnant women. The result was that in three years (1959–1962) 8,000 children throughout the world were born without limbs. The steroidal hormones estrogen and progestin have been discovered to be possible causes of birth defects, including limb and heart abnormalities. (For a discussion of the medical use of these, see Chapter 8.) Both estrogen and progestin were formerly used to prevent miscarriage. Progestins were also used in a pregnancy test. The general rule now is that a woman should avoid any pregnancy test that involves taking hormones. Use of hormones to avert miscarriage is unjustified, in the opinion of the Food and Drug Administration. In the 1950s the estrogenic hormone diethylstilbestrol (DES) was freely given to prevent miscarriage and has been found responsible for a rare form of vaginal cancer in girls and some genital abnormalities in boys whose mothers were given the drug during pregnancy.

Other prescription drugs that can have bad effects on the unborn include:

• Barbiturates. Heavy use in pregnancy can result in an addicted baby.

• Amphetamines. Used as "uppers" and as help in weight loss, these drugs can cause birth defects.

• "Minor" tranquilizers and other medications of the meprobamate or benzodiazepine types, when taken in early pregnancy, increase risk of cleft lip and cleft palate in the baby.

• Aspirin and other drugs containing salicylate should not be taken during the last three months of pregnancy except under medical supervision. They can prolong labor and cause excessive bleeding.

If you've grown accustomed to using drugstore remedies for a cold, a cough, a minor allergy flare-up, or occasional nervousness or insomnia, it's a good idea to toss all these nonprescription helpers into the wastebasket before you enter pregnancy. They really are drugs, even though they don't require a doctor's prescription. Hundreds of liquid medications contain high percentages of alcohol. What's more, because pregnancy may aggravate minor aches and pains, you could find yourself taking a good deal more medication than usual, at considerable increase in risk to you and your baby. *The bottom line on drugs and pregnancy.* Don't take anything on your own. Take only drugs that your own physician prescribes. If you go to a different doctor for any reason, be sure that doctor knows you're pregnant or trying to become pregnant.

Nutrition and Pregnancy

> *If she happens to desire clay, chalk, or coals (as many pregnant women do), give her beans boiled with sugar; and if she happens to long for any thing she cannot obtain, let her drink a large draught of pure cold water.*
>
> *When she is not far from her labour, let her eat every day seven roasted figs before her meat, and sometimes let her lick a little honey.*
>
> —*From* The Master-Piece

Gone are the days, we feel sure, when pregnant women were firmly told to restrain their eating and gain no more than fifteen or seventeen pounds during pregnancy in order to avoid a fat baby, a fat mother and possible birth complications.

Nutrition and obstetric experts now agree—and support it with enormous amounts of research—that "eating for two" is best; more precisely, eating *wisely* for two. Under the best nutritional conditions, a woman of average prepregnancy height and weight will gain between twenty-five and thirty pounds by the time she delivers her child. Some perfectly normal women may gain either more or less.

You will probably gain little or no weight in the first few weeks following conception. You might even lose weight. But near the end of the third month you will normally have a steady weight gain that remains just about constant right up to birth—about a pound, or slightly less, each week.

Pregnancy is no time for dieting, in terms of losing fat. If you think you have a few unwanted pounds at the time you begin pregnancy, best to forget about them until after the baby comes.

Even with the considerable weight gain, good nutrition in pregnancy will not leave you fat afterward. All the required nutrients—calories, protein, minerals and vitamins—have a job to do. Again speaking in terms of average sizes, almost half of the weight gained at full term under ideal conditions goes to the fetus and its biological furniture, the placenta and amniotic fluid. The mother's share of the weight gain will include additional blood volume, body fluid, added uterus and breast tissue, and some fatty tissue. Obviously a good deal of this will be lost at childbirth. You may have a minimal amount of weight to lose later; if you breast-feed your child, you will probably postpone reducing until weaning.

What foods to eat, and how much? (See the charts in Chapter 2.) And equip yourself with an authoritative handbook on nutrition that includes pregnancy nutrition. Your physician's office can possibly supply one. The National Academy of Sciences–National Research Council's handbook *Recommended Dietary Allowances* is one of the excellent guides. It provides background on what nutrients you need and what foods are good sources of them.

If your prepregnancy diet has been adequate—around 2,100 calories daily if you're within an average weight range—you'll probably add about 300 calories a day, or about 15 percent, for pregnancy. If you've been getting about 45 grams of protein daily, it's recommended that you add another 30 grams—a hefty protein increase. In practice, you can take care of both increased requirements—of calories and protein—by adding a good three cupfuls of skim milk to your regular daily diet. You can vary this by using cottage cheese, yogurt, lean meat, fish and chicken, all excellent protein sources with relatively modest calorie counts.

Women who get cramps and diarrhea from milk and milk products need special dietary counseling in pregnancy in order to get adequate supplies of protein and calcium. Women who are vegetarians also need special diet planning in pregnancy. They may require supplementary zinc, chromium and vitamin B_{12} (which isn't found in plants), as well as iron.

Don't restrict salt during pregnancy unless so directed by your doctor. Drink lots of fluids.

SUPPLEMENTS

You should consult with your physician as well as relying on your own views and customary practices regarding your vitamin and mineral needs in pregnancy. There are excellent vitamin-mineral supplements designed especially for pregnancy that your physician may recommend to ensure an adequate supply should your diet fall short. Many doctors will hasten to add that vitamin supplements are no substitute for good diet planning—only an added insurance policy.

One supplement recommended for all pregnant women is iron; food sources cannot satisfy the demand for great increases in iron needed to keep red blood cells properly oxygenated and to handle the greatly increased amount of blood circulating in you and your unborn child. As you can see on the charts in Chapter 2 and will hear from your physician, from 30 to 60 milligrams of extra iron each day should be standard practice during pregnancy and for some months afterward.

The vitamin component folate, or folic acid, may be recommended as a supplement, though not all authorities agree on this. Severe deficiency of this vitamin is associated with megaloblastic anemia, a serious disease. Added folate in tablet form can protect women under some medications, those with chronic disease, and those with closely spaced pregnancies.

Exercise During Pregnancy: Body Building Both Ways

You will want to continue your favorite sports if you are already an exercise fan. If you're not an exerciser, consider starting a fitness routine that will benefit you and your baby. Physically fit women have been observed to have easier births and fewer complications.

Pregnant women just starting on an exercise routine should have a medical evaluation, including stress tests. Your physician may administer the tests or may refer you to a specialist (such as a physical therapist) who does this kind of testing and evaluation.

Your work capacity—a measurable index—is lower during the first trimester of pregnancy, a fact that may comfort you if you feel weak and helpless during that stage. During the second trimester you may be able to do physical work at your nonpregnant level— if the effort is not affected by body weight, such as cycling or swimming. Weight-influenced exertion, including walking, jogging, tennis and cross-country skiing, will naturally take more effort as your weight increases. Remember also that your body's center of gravity shifts greatly—you're carrying many extra pounds out in front and below the waist—which can compromise your balance. Most doctors rule out highly competitive sports in advanced pregnancy; and let's face it, if competition is important to you, you're quite likely to lose in these circumstances.

Unless you're a highly skilled jogger, you face risk of injury if you continue jogging vigorously during pregnancy. The bouncing motion puts strain on abdominal muscles, hips, knees and ankles. Sports experts recommend that you consider switching to walking, cycling or swimming.

If your heart is set on continuing your favorite exercise or training program, and it is one of the weight-influenced ones, consider decreasing the work by stages, as your pregnancy and weight advance. Alternating work and rest, or jogging and walking, can help you stay trim without the burden of fatigue.

Training for Childbirth

Ferdinand Lamaze, a French doctor, inadvertently started the wave of childbirth preparation courses in this country when an American woman he had in one of his classes returned to America and wrote a book about her experience. Now an estimated 30 percent of prospective American parents take some kind of training in preparation for childbirth.

Training techniques differ, but most include breathing, pushing and relaxation exercises aimed at working with, not against, the body in expelling the infant. Most courses call for active support and assistance from a personal partner or "coach," who may be the pregnant woman's spouse, relative or friend, and who will assist during the actual labor and delivery. Most courses also include a psychological dimension, intended to overcome fear and diminish pain.

Lamaze-based courses usually consist of six two-hour sessions, attended once a week from about the seventh month of pregnancy. Instructors are health professionals, often registered nurses, most of whom have had at least one child by the Lamaze method and who have also had considerable obstetrical training. Attending these classes, you and your coach/partner will learn a good deal about the parturition (childbirth) process, the timing of contractions, and the breathing and muscular techniques that work best during the various stages of labor (and also keep the two of you busy, which helps).

Critics of childbirth preparation courses fear some classes are operated by high-pressure enthusiasts who evangelize "the method" and claim there is no such thing as pain in labor. In the event of a birth complication requiring Caesarean surgery or in contractions severe enough to require pain relievers, the mother may feel she has failed "the method" and serious emotional reactions could result.

Not so, according to two of the national organizations for child-birth training. Instead, the idea behind these courses is *prepared* birth, so that whatever happens, including serious complications, the mother and her partner understand and can take part in managing events.

Fetal Monitoring

Use of an electronic instrument for keeping watch on the progress of labor and the state of the unborn child is in medical controversy as this is written. The device consists of electrodes at first attached to the mother's belly, and as labor goes on, to the scalp of the unborn fetus. A flickering monitor screen displays an oscilloscopic picture of the duration and intensity of uterine contractions, and a beeping instrument amplifies the fetal heartbeat. The monitor is designed to extend, if not replace, the traditional monitoring by nurse and physician attending the birth. The electronic device is intended to capture any signals of fetal distress sooner than they would be seen by medical attendants, so that any needed intervention, such as Caesarean surgery, can be started at once. Some obstetricians believe fetal monitoring ought to be a standard practice in hospital delivery services.

Those physicians who oppose routine fetal monitoring say that possibly more babies would be saved by early intervention with surgery, but that more mothers would die because the Caesarean section, which is major surgery, carries a greater statistical risk to the mother than does vaginal delivery. They believe monitoring leads to unnecessary Caesarean surgery in some cases, and that attaching instruments can harm the mother and child. With monitoring, there is a slightly increased risk of infection.

Another objection to fetal monitoring is that it depersonalizes the birth process, with the woman restrained on the table and hooked up to instruments, and with the steady beeping sound and the shifting images on the screen. A change in the beep might frighten the mother into thinking something terrible is about to happen; and fear may interfere with the normal labor process. But other women are greatly reassured by the sights and sounds of monitoring, especially those who have had birth preparation training and whose partner is present.

Ask your obstetrician whether fetal monitoring is available, optional or routine in the facility where you'll give birth. If it is any of these, ask for more information on what it does and what its benefits are, so that together you and your doctor can make an informed decision whether you need it, or want it, and whether you will be in a hospital where your wishes will be accommodated.

Realize also that whatever you and your physician may plan will perhaps have to be changed. If you planned no monitoring, assuming a normal labor, complications may make a monitor essential; conversely, a smooth labor on a busy day may *not* be monitored if high-risk patients need all the available equipment.

Prenatal Diagnostic Tests

Amniocentesis is a quick, almost painless procedure for obtaining a sample of the amniotic fluid, which surrounds the fetus. After determining the position of the fetus and placenta, often with ultrasound monitoring, the surgeon uses a long needle to enter the uterus through the abdominal wall. The test has a high degree of safety, according to clinical experts. It's extremely unlikely that the needle is going to touch the baby; the test is made when the uterus is quite well developed and the fetus can—and usually does—bounce away if it's near the entering needle. (A small possibility of fetal injury or infection does exist, however. For this reason, amniocentesis should be done only for valid medical reasons.)

What can such a prenatal test tell you? The amniotic fluid, a remarkable substance, reflects many genetic and biochemical conditions that can be accurately assessed. Among them:

1. Tay-Sachs disease, a devastating condition that mainly strikes people of East European Jewish ancestry. It causes progressive nerve deterioration and apparent great suffering and is invariably lethal to the child in babyhood or early childhood.
2. Sickle-cell anemia, a disease of misshapen red blood cells that causes disability and early death. It runs predominantly in black families.
3. Cooley's anemia, or thalassemia, an inherited blood disease that may affect people of Mediterranean ancestry.
4. Chromosomal abnormality, such as Down's syndrome, the cause of mental retardation and heart defects, may run in some families and also has a strikingly higher incidence among children born to older mothers. It is standard practice today to recommend amniocentesis for all pregnant women above age 35.

Besides the genetic conditions that can be diagnosed by amniocentesis, cell tests of the amniotic fluid can render biochemical information about the stage of fetal development and other factors. When, for medical reasons, an early delivery is considered, a truly important piece of information is whether the infant lungs are sufficiently developed for survival. Precise testing for surfactant, or surface-acting substance, in the amniotic fluid reveals whether the fetal lungs are mature enough to function in the outside atmosphere.

Amniocentesis allows the option of either continuing the pregnancy or, if the fetus is severely affected, having a therapeutic abortion. It also allows opportunity for parenthood to people formerly unwilling to attempt pregnancy because of genetic risks in their families. Now they can learn whether a fetus is normal and can be carried to term, and more and more women are taking advantage of this option. Most encouraging is the fact that even though they're being tested because there is some risk of fetal abnormality, about 97 percent of the test results are negative—the fetus is normal and healthy.

You may wish to learn about and consider genetic counseling and testing if you are pregnant and:

- Are over 35
- Have already had an affected child
- Have had affected members in your family or the child's father's family

Ultrasonography is a technique that projects an image of the interior structures of the body by directing inaudible, superswift sound waves inside the body. It can tell the diagnostic expert the fetal size, age, and exact location and position inside the uterus. In many cases the sonogram can show physical deformities, such as spinal defects. Sonography can be of immense help in establishing the stage of fetal development. Because it gives direct visualization, it's useful as a guide during amniocentesis. It's specially helpful for detecting twins when other fetal signals are confusing. Because sonography is painless, doesn't give off radiation, does not invade the body and is believed to have no effects on the tissues through which it passes, scientific investigators predict it will be used for more and more diagnostic procedures in the future—many of them related to pregnancy and childbirth.

Maternal AFP Blood Testing. Levels of alpha-fetoprotein in the mother's blood can point to possible neural tube abnormalities, the most common birth defect in this country (with the exception of heart disorders). This defect represents a lapse or interruption during a critical phase of spinal-cord development. It may cause spinabifida, or open spine (an abnormal division between the vertebrae), leading to fetal death for many and severe disability for those who survive birth. It may also cause anencephaly, developmental failure in brain and skull, which is invariably fatal.

The newly developed AFP blood test is not as sensitive as amniocentesis for detecting neural tube defects, but because it is rapid and inexpensive it may become a routine way to locate such problems among pregnant women with no apparent risk factors. If AFP blood testing becomes a screening routine for all pregnant women, those with positive signals can be referred for amniocentesis testing, for a more specific diagnosis.

Your Baby's Sex

Many prospective parents have some degree of preference for either a girl or a boy. In the past there have been many cases where parents had such a powerful preference that the child who was not the "right" sex grew up under a cruel burden of being a disappointment, of trying to fill both sex roles or of rejecting his or her own gender.

If you have amniocentesis, you can learn whether your baby will be a boy or girl—if you want to know. Your genetic counselor will gladly withhold the information if you'd rather be surprised. The writer Nora Ephron has said that when she and her former husband, Carl Bernstein, voted to be told, they were at first thrilled, and then experienced a curious depression and letdown. Why? Not because their first child was going to be a boy, but because the knowledge of it deprived them of half their fantasies about the unborn child. Before the baby comes, you may need your dreams about both a girl and a boy; you may, in effect, lose one dream-child if you learn a baby's sex in advance.

Genetic research projects now are being aimed at parents' choosing the sex of a child before conception. Some efforts concentrate on the timing of the ovulatory cycle, early or late, as a determinant. A method involving acid or alkaline douches has so far not yielded significant results. Newer techniques are being worked on to separate X-bearing from Y-bearing sperm in the father's semen. The sex is determined at the moment of fertilization by whether the single sperm reaching the ovum carries the X chromosome (for a girl) or the Y chromosome (for a boy). Laboratory scientists are trying to find differences in sperm behavior—Y-bearing sperm are said to swim faster—in order to inseminate the prospective mother with semen carrying predominantly the preferred sperm type.

Ahead of Time

Babies can—and often do—arrive spontaneously well before their gestation period is complete. After seven months, chances for survival are good. Survival rates are improving because of strides recently made in hospital intensive care nurseries (ICNs). The premature baby usually has to overcome low birth weight and may be threatened by breathing problems (medically termed "respiratory distress syndrome," or RDS) because of its immature lungs.

Early delivery is sometimes deliberately scheduled because of medical conditions. These may include previous obstetric problems or illness of the mother (particularly kidney problems). At one time the babies of diabetic mothers were routinely delivered early to prevent birth complications, but today such babies may often be carried to term, thanks to fetal and maternal monitoring techniques. And in some cases there's an unexpected emergency condition that requires the doctor to either induce labor with drugs or perform a Caesarean section.

It was once considered rather fashionable for mothers to have medically induced early delivery, purely for convenience or to shorten the tedious waiting. Today medical authorities believe that full term is best unless there's a pressing medical reason for early delivery. When there is, tests for fetal maturity can now be made, and delivery can be electronically monitored, so the early-arriving child can be brought forth with increased safety and confidence.

The Caesarean Section

Caesarean surgery got its name from the time-honored notion that the Roman emperor Julius Caesar (100–44 B.C.) was delivered through an abdominal incision. But Dr. Ernest Klein, author of the *Comprehensive Etymological Dictionary of the English Language,* doubts this, pointing out that Caesar's mother was alive and well during her son's reign. At that time, abdominal delivery was never performed on a living woman, but only as an effort to rescue a baby inside a woman who had just died.

The Caesarean surgical procedure (also called C-section) is done in an estimated half-million births each year in this country. Although it is major surgery, which means there are always some risks, the C-section can be a real boon in a number of conditions. Among the perfectly valid reasons to consider Caesarean birth are a too small pelvic opening for vaginal delivery; failure of labor to progress properly, with danger that the child will be oxygen-deprived; having the fetus in the wrong position, such as a breech presentation; a disease of the mother, such as diabetes, that might endanger her in a vaginal delivery; a disease that might endanger the baby, such as an active herpesvirus infection; and previous Caesarean births that may have weakened or damaged the uterine walls.

However, the "once a Caesarean, always a Caesarean" rule no longer holds fast. Often physicians will allow a woman to have a vaginal delivery even after a previous Caesarean, provided the current labor is normal and proceeds smoothly.

The major statistical risk to the child born by Caesarean surgery is prematurity, usually in cases where the operation is scheduled before labor starts. Tests of amniotic fluid to determine fetal lung maturity reduce a great deal of this risk.

The possible complications to mothers undergoing Caesarean surgery include hemorrhage, infections, blood clots and possible internal injuries—risks similar to those of any major abdominal operation. In recent years these operative risks have been greatly reduced; they are mentioned here to point out that C-section is not, as is sometimes assumed, an easy way to avoid labor pains.

When something unforeseen dictates childbirth by Caesarean surgery, a mother who has prepared for and expects to take part in delivery and to have immediate contact with her baby may be bitterly disappointed and feel she has failed in the most important job of all. Of course this isn't so.

Birthplace Choices

At the beginning of this century, births almost invariably took place in the home. On the other hand, a short generation ago giving birth was almost always a standardized, well-anesthetized hospital procedure over which the mother and father had little control and the infant was hustled off into the nursery. Today, in great part because of demands by women's and consumers' organizations, you may choose from a variety of birthing facilities to meet your personal needs and wishes.

With more than a quarter of parents-to-be attending childbirth preparation courses and expecting to participate totally, this need is being met by many hospital maternity wings as well as by newer "birthing rooms." These are comfortable places with homelike furnishings and sometimes kitchenettes. Labor, delivery and rooming-in all take place here. Equipment for any possible emergency is near at hand, but isn't evident in the living/birthing quarters. Such lying-in facilities, called alternative birth centers, offer a big change from standard hospital routines, in which the father paced corridors while the delivering mother was moved from labor room to delivery room to recovery room, and eventually to her hospital room, sometimes not seeing her baby for hours after the birth.

Much more often nowadays, fathers have been trained and are allowed to assist during labor and delivery, the mother is permitted to hold and nurse her child immediately, newborns room with their mothers, and sometimes brothers and sisters are allowed to visit.

The process of "bonding"—giving the newborn baby prompt eye and body contact with its mother—has the support and approval of the American Medical Association. Helping the new baby feel at home in the world—as well as helping the mother to be close to her new child—is such a commendable idea that one wonders why the impersonal, superefficient routines of fifteen or twenty years ago were ever allowed to prevail.

The LeBoyer method of delivery, named for the French obstetrician, Dr. Frédéric LeBoyer, author of *Birth without Violence,* was designed to welcome the new baby with the utmost comfort and gentleness, keeping things as warm, dark and quiet as possible, sparing the child the customary shocks of the delivery process. Room lights are kept low instead of glaring (the obstetrical staff may use spotlights for needed visualization). Music and low voices are heard in preference to noisy machinery and equipment. The newborn baby is gently lowered into a warm bath, as soothing as the amniotic fluid from which it came. The baby is then placed on the mother's body as soon as possible. Today a good many obstetricians use some or most of these techniques for handling the newborn.

Within the past few years, increasing numbers of mothers have chosen to deliver at home. Home-birth organizations have grown throughout the country, providing instruction and procedures for giving birth at home, assisted by a physician or a midwife or both. Most—but not all—doctors strongly recommend that the delivery take place within reach of hospital emergency facilities. They point out that in cases of fetal distress there is seldom time enough to move a woman in labor to the hospital.

The trend toward home birth influenced the development of new facilities in hospitals, which are now moving toward providing both the comforts of home and the technology of the medical center. This trend promises safer, happier delivery for both the mother and the baby, and much more participation by the whole family.

After you have become pregnant, you will want to learn all about the types of childbirth services and facilities available to you, so make plans with your obstetrician's help. Then discuss the places to consider for the event with your childbirth-course director, and make your final decisions after consulting your spouse and perhaps other family members.

7

PREGNANCY CONTROLS: CONTRACEPTIVES, STERILIZATION AND ABORTION

At the beginning of this century, a fertile woman's babies came tumbling one after another, often at considerable risk of health both to the woman and to successive infants born to a worn-out, child-ridden mother. The growing control over pregnancy has provided women opportunities to develop themselves individually as well as to achieve a successful family life.

By permitting planning, control of the reproductive function benefits the family. Children are more likely to get a full share of parents' time and attention during infancy; fathers and mothers can better manage budgets, careers and other interests. Increasing numbers of women today are postponing first babies until their thirties —an extended childbearing span made safer by improved prenatal care, childbirth training and diagnostic testing techniques such as amniocentesis and ultrasonography.

In this chapter we will examine the principal methods of fertility control: contraceptives, sterilization and abortion. We will discuss the various contraceptive measures and their relative safety and effectiveness. We will describe sterilization procedures for both men and women to show the options available to those who want to make fertility control permanent. Finally, we will talk about abortion, the various ways it is performed and the length of gestation involved in each method.

Women of all cultures and throughout recorded time have used just about every means imaginable to prevent pregnancy. They drank potions made from gunpowder, mercury, camel saliva and reproductive organs of animals. They inserted plugs in their vaginas made of wool, lint, oiled paper or beeswax; some were soaked in dung, oil, honey, wine or fruit juice. Incantations and the wearing of talismans were thought to be helpful. Perhaps they were, but folklore rarely recounts the failures.

Male contraceptive devices go back in history too. The first sheath for the penis, made of linen, was said to have been designed in the 1500s by Gabriel Fallopius, the famed anatomist whose name was given to our uterine tubes. But he wasn't seeking to spare women from conception; he was trying to protect men from venereal infection.

Later, in the mid-1700s, the skin, or gut sheath, came into use. Our usual term, the condom, is believed to be a slight distortion of the name of the inventor, Dr. Condon. At the start of the twentieth century, condoms were made from rubber; hence the term "rubber" in referring to the condom.

Birth Control in America: A Sorry Story

Our present freedom in matters of birth control hasn't been achieved without a number of battles along the way. In 1873 Anthony Comstock, a self-appointed anti-vice crusader hustled a piece of legislation through a compliant or indifferent Congress that the righteous felt would protect morality by making it a criminal offense to possess or mail pornographic pictures and publications. But Comstock's personal definition of obscenity, as written into the law, included "any article of medicine for the prevention of conception."

Following this, Comstock and his road company of zealots traveled through the country, coercing every state legislature (with the exception of New Mexico) into passing obscenity laws that would restrict contraceptive information or supplies. In Connecticut, even the private use of contraceptives was a crime punishable by fine or imprisonment.

The Comstock Act meant that physicians could not, on pain of imprisonment, order textbooks that carried scientific information on contraception. Professional journals could not refer to birth control in any way. Physicians began challenging this restriction, and in 1912 the president of the American Medical Association made clear the stand of organized medicine when he declared that contraception "benefits the parents, it is decidedly beneficial to society, and it is even more merciful to the unborn and unconceived creature which it frequently saves from a life of misery."

During this particularly wretched stretch in women's history, wives not only were expected to be compliant to their husbands' sexual wishes while not having any of their own, but at the same time were denied any measure of birth control. No wonder the habitual "wifely headache" found its way into American tradition. Even more helpless, but not by much, were the unmarried women who became pregnant.

By 1916 Margaret Sanger, an American nurse, had become so enraged at the sickness, exhaustion and deaths she saw from botched abortions among constantly pregnant poor women that she openly set up a birth-control clinic to instruct women in such methods of contraception as were known at the time. For this, she was arrested and jailed. Supporters, including doctors who risked arrest and loss of their licenses, rose to her defense, and a long series of court actions, petitions and resolutions favoring legal contraceptive advice ensued. Legal statutes regarding contraception did not, however, become even relatively free of shackles until well into the 1950s.

Of the many pregnancy control methods, none is perfect, safe and effective for everybody, but for each woman there is a contraceptive plan that is best for *her*.

There are some primary factors you should consider and evaluate when choosing a contraceptive method, product or device:

• *Safety,* which means freedom from risking your health or your life.

• *Effectiveness* in preventing conception. Since most methods work almost all of the time if they're used exactly according to directions, this means evaluating your own lifestyle, personality and habits and deciding which method suits you best.

• *Convenience,* another highly personal factor that includes considerations of which method is easiest and most pleasant for you to use, your and your partner's sensitivities, and the need for spontaneity in your sex life.

Contraceptive Methods and Non-Methods

Here are a few approaches to avoiding conception, briefly described to show that contraceptive efforts are not entirely limited to substances and devices. Anything that might interfere with the union of sperm and ovum can be consciously employed as a contraceptive measure. Some of these practices include:

• *Abstinence.* For moral, religious or personal reasons, many young women choose not to become sexually active until marriage. Today's increased candor about sexual expression, with greater freedom in sexual activity, leads a great many of these young persons to fear their choice of postponement means something is wrong with them. There isn't.

Teen-agers who have been sexually active may decide to look for the "right" monogamous relationship. Others fear this may be a sign of impaired sexual health. It isn't. It's perfectly normal, and may be a sign of developing emotional maturity.

During much of the past century and well into the current one, married women could avoid pregnancy by pretending chronic ill health, a state that justified curtailing sexual activities. This was, alas, the only recourse many women had, but clearly, it caused more problems than it avoided.

Finally, planned periodic abstinence, which limits intercourse to times when a mature egg is not likely to be available for fertilization, is the classical practice most widely known as the "rhythm method." The Human Life and Natural Family Planning Foundation backs the training of couples to recognize signs of the woman's fertility and practice sexual abstinence during the fertile times of her cycle. The method takes into account the body temperature (which rises near the time of ovulation), the cycling of menstrual blood, and the changes in cervical mucus (wet during fertile phases). Women also learn to detect various body signals associated with ovulation, such as increased breast tenderness, water retention, the usually mild abdominal pain called *Mittelschmerz,* and even mood swings that have no basis other than hormonal changes associated with ovulation.

Used alone, the calendar, temperature and mucus methods have high failure rates. But used in combination, and with determination and discipline, they give results that adherents of natural family planning regard as highly satisfactory. The necessary abstinence of up to ten days each month may serve to reinforce emotional bonds between man and woman and promote mutual understanding and responsibility.

Natural family planning, to be successful, requires high motivation, careful record keeping, patience and extensive training. In her book *Natural Sex,* Mary Shivanandan points out that anyone who wants to master the natural methods, either to achieve or to avoid pregnancy, ought to find a qualified teacher or program. (Referral service is offered by the Human Life and Natural Family Planning Foundation in Washington, D.C.) It's not a system to be learned from a book, she says—not even her book.

• *Coitus interruptus,* withdrawal of the penis from the vagina before ejaculation, and *coitus reservatus,* suppression of ejaculation, are time-honored practices for preventing sperm from entering the vagina or the cervical canal. Failure rates are high.

• *Douching.* Flushing out the vagina with water or a disinfectant solution, done promptly after intercourse, is still widely employed as a contraceptive measure. It is totally unreliable. Sperm can reach the cervix within 90 seconds after ejaculation, so washing semen out of the vagina later on is usually of no help at all in preventing conception.

Contraceptives: How to Choose, How to Use

BARRIERS

Condoms and diaphragms are the most widely used among "barrier" contraceptives. Doctors usually classify spermicides—foams, creams and jellies—as barrier methods too, because they physically block as well as kill sperm. We will discuss them in connection with, as well as separately from, the inert devices that serve as dams keeping semen away from the cervix.

• *Condoms,* or sheaths (also called prophylactics, safes, rubbers), are today made of thin rubber or of lamb's intestinal membrane. Condoms are easy to carry (they fit in a pocket, purse or wallet), easy to buy, and inexpensive. They are available without a prescription and can be used without medical instruction. In many states they're displayed right beside the cash register in drugstores and supermarkets, permitting a discreet purchase. Contrary to the common belief that only men buy condoms, marketing surveys show that 25 percent of them are purchased by women. Besides the more costly and comparatively more luxurious "skin" condoms, there are latex, or rubber, condoms of varying thinness, different colors and several textures. Some are prelubricated. Rubber and latex condoms are dated on the package as insurance against deterioration from age. In addition, you should store them in a cool place; heat can cause rubber to break down.

According to family-planning experts, the barrier contraceptive methods, including condoms, are about 97 percent effective in preventing conception *if they're used correctly and consistently.* This is about the same effectiveness rating as that for the pill or the IUD. Unfortunately, field statistics indicate that of every 100 women relying on her partner's condom protection only, anywhere from 3 to 36 will become pregnant in a year's time.

It is possible to use condoms and be confident of almost total effectiveness, but this takes skill: you must be careful to prevent the sheath from rupturing, slipping off in use, and spilling semen at the top. For total effectiveness, a new sheath must be used for every single act of intercourse.

To accommodate the volume and pressure of ejaculation, space should be left at the tip of the condom as it is rolled onto the erected penis. It is also a good idea to squeeze an inch or so of spermicidal jelly or a small blob of foam in the center of the condom before it is put on. Soon after ejaculation the sheathed penis should be withdrawn, with the top edge of the sheath held firmly to prevent spilling any semen. If the condom rips or slips off during use, the woman should use vaginal foam immediately.

• *The cervical diaphragm,* a disk-shaped rubber barrier, is slipped

BIRTH CONTROL METHODS

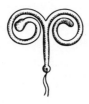 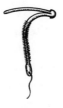 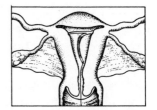

Inert plastic IUDs (such as the coil shown at left) probably work by causing uterine tissue reaction. The copper-containing IUDs (such as the Copper 7 pictured in the center) are wrapped with thin copper wire in order to promote mild tissue reaction. On the right, an IUD is shown in position within the uterus with top bar across upper space, stem of "7" toward neck of cervix, and only the string left outside the cervical opening.

 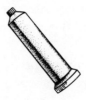 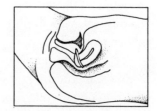

Typical diaphragm (left) *has spring inside rolled-rubber edge and may be round or oval. Spermicidal gel or cream* (center) *should be used liberally on inside surface and edges. In place* (right), *diaphragm slips beneath pubic bone in front, covers cervical opening at back. Cervical opening can be felt through diaphragm.*

 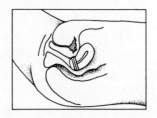

Cervical cap (left) *fits snugly over cervix* (right) *and usually must be removed for menstrual period. But new test models may have one-way valve permitting menstrual flow to escape.*

inside the vagina, where it lies braced between the pubic bone and the back wall of the vaginal space, covering the cervical opening. As with the condom, a small spoonful of spermicidal jelly or foam is placed in the diaphragm before insertion. Diaphragms are coming back into style, particularly with younger women who want to avoid oral contraceptives and IUDs and with "over thirty" women who have used the pill for several years and believe it's time to stop.

Diaphragms are prescribed and usually fitted by a doctor, though trained technicians and nurses do a good share of diaphragm fitting too. At the fitting, you will get instruction and practice in placing it properly, and in its proper use and maintenance. If the diaphragm is inserted incorrectly, it may leave the cervix exposed to semen, with the risk of pregnancy increased by the fact that you think you're safe.

Because the diaphragm is inserted before intercourse, it usually takes a certain amount of foresight and planning—unless, of course, you want to put it in immediately before coitus. One possible advantage of the diaphragm over the condom is that there's no need to interrupt love play while a sheath is put on. But there are exceptions to these presumed drawbacks. The late Alan Guttmacher, M.D., president of Planned Parenthood for many years, recalled that he once asked a patient the secret of her success in using a diaphragm over many years with no failures. "Tell me in your own words just how you put in the diaphragm," he said, "then I'll be able to explain it better to other patients." The woman looked somewhat embarrassed and said, "Well, to tell you the truth, I've never put it in myself. My husband has always put it in."

Diaphragms come in sizes from 2½ to 4½ inches in diameter. This range does not indicate anything about the capacity of your vagina or uterus—it's simply the distance between the back wall, where the rim rests, and the front wall, where the opposite side of the rim fits against the pelvic bone. Because these anatomical dimensions can be altered by pregnancy and childbirth, it's important to be refitted for a diaphragm when you resume contraception after having a baby. Periodically, hold your diaphragm up to a good light and check for any possible pinpoint-size holes; they occur rarely, but if they do, could allow passage of sperm. It's also recommended to have your diaphragm size rechecked each year, as well as after any weight change of ten pounds or more, and following abortion.

Professionals who work in family-planning clinics—doctors, nurses, counselors and administrators—choose barrier contraceptives for themselves in much greater percentages than does the general population, a survey reveals. They also use the double protection of spermicide cream, foam or jelly along with either condom or diaphragm. The combination method provides very effective contraception without the side effects or safety risks of the pill and IUDs.

The major barrier contraceptive methods have some bonuses and possible drawbacks:

• Condoms offer protection against venereal infection; indeed, they were originally devised for just that purpose. There's also some evidence that spermicidal foams and jellies give some protection by killing infectious organisms (but they shouldn't be relied on for this purpose).

• Common complaints against condoms include loss of sensitivity (as compared to no covering at all), risk of rupturing, and as we mentioned, interruption of foreplay in order to put on the sheath. The range of styles and thinness now available can overcome a great percentage of sensitivity complaints.

• All barrier methods are local; they don't affect the whole body system. They can't cause cramps, as the IUD can, or cause the risk of circulatory mishaps, which are attributed to the pill.

Research now being conducted indicates a possible risk in using talcum powder for dusting condoms or diaphragms. Particles of talc and asbestos-like fibers have been found in ovarian tumors, raising the suspicion that talc may migrate from the vagina into the tubes leading to the ovaries. The safest course is to avoid using anything in the vagina that might contain talc.

SPERMICIDES

You can use foam, cream or jelly spermicides alone, without a diaphragm or condom. These products can be purchased at the drugstore without a prescription and are easy and pleasant to use.

They are somewhat less effective against conception, statistically speaking, than combinations of spermicide plus a condom or a diaphragm. Aerosol foams are rated higher in effectiveness than are jellies and creams. But as with many other contraceptive methods, used correctly and for every sexual episode, spermicide products are highly effective. You must use the foam, cream or jelly one hour or less before intercourse, and if you want to douche later, you should wait six to eight hours after intercourse.

Vaginal tablets that produce foam on contact with genital moisture are gaining in popularity and at the foaming stage are just as effective as other foam spermicides. Sometimes a user doesn't have enough vaginal fluid to build up the foam, and the fizzing action of the spermicide may produce a sensation of heat.

If you prefer a waxy vaginal suppository, there are several easy-to-use varieties available over the counter. But do read labels; only a few vaginal suppositories are for purposes of contraception. Of those that are, timing is important for effective use. The waxy tablet must be inserted fifteen minutes before intercourse. If placed earlier, it can become ineffective. If placed later—just before intercourse—the tablet doesn't have time to melt and therefore may not work.

THE IUD

Intrauterine devices are small plastic or metal gadgets with a string attached. The IUD is put inside the uterus by a doctor, who slips the device through the cervical canal into its proper location, with the string left extending through the mouth of the cervix. The string is important, because it will indicate that the IUD is still in place when you have subsequent pelvic examinations. If you choose the convenience of the IUD, keep track of it. From time to time, feel for the string to be sure it still protrudes from your cervix.

At this writing there are about half a dozen types of IUDs on the market in this country. They come in various shapes, such as 7s, Ts, loops and coils, and in different sizes. The IUD's presence inside the uterus interferes with a fertilized egg's getting a toehold on the walls. Some IUDs are made of inert materials, but two kinds also emit minute amounts of either copper or the hormone progesterone and provide biochemical action as well. Copper-bearing IUDs need to be replaced every three years. Progesterone-containing ones need replacing every year.

The IUD is convenient (you don't have to remember to do anything), unobtrusive (neither sex partner is aware of the IUD during coitus) and effective (in practice, a 1 to 6 percent failure rate). After the IUD is inserted there's no care needed, other than to report to your doctor for a yearly checkup.

But the IUD is not the perfect contraceptive for all women. Some women have menstrual cramps and heavy menstrual flow when using an IUD. These problems can be severe enough to require removal of the device. In addition, should the IUD be expelled from the uterus without your knowing it, you could be unprotected and risk pregnancy. With IUDs, there is an increased risk of ectopic pregnancy, which means a fetus growing somewhere outside the uterus, usually in a Fallopian tube. This requires immediate medical attention, so should you miss a period while wearing an IUD, get a medical checkup promptly. Do not use a home-pregnancy test; such tests are not dependable in a tubal pregnancy.

IUDs have sometimes been found to perforate the uterine tissues and even migrate into the intestinal cavity. Such cases are rare, but they are of course quite serious and require surgery.

Some conditions may rule out using the IUD. If you have once had any of the following, discuss them thoroughly with your doctor before having an IUD inserted:

- Cancer or any other disorder of uterus or cervix
- Regularly heavy menstrual flow
- Severe menstrual cramps
- Spotting between periods
- Any gynecologic infections, including VD
- Recent pregnancy, abortion or miscarriage
- Surgery in the genital area
- Allergy to copper, or disordered copper metabolism
- Anemia
- Attacks of faintness or weakness
- Heart conditions
- Coagulation defects (clotting problems)

IUD User's Check List

Here are some points to remember before using the IUD:

• You may consider having the IUD inserted during your menstrual period. This way, both you and your doctor are assured that you're not pregnant at the time.

• It's important for IUD insertion to be done by someone who is both experienced and comfortable with the procedure. This could be your private physician. In a clinic, a trained paraprofessional may do insertions.

• Whoever your insertion specialist is, discuss with him the type of IUD you should use. Be sure you understand why a given device is the best one for you.

• Expect some cramping and spotting right after insertion; if you don't have either, fine. But if you develop sharp pains and if you can feel a knob instead of a string at the opening of your cervix, go back to your doctor or clinic.

• For the first two months or so, check your underwear and the water in the toilet for signs of blood.

• Heavier menstrual periods after IUD insertion are common. But if bleeding seems excessive, return for a checkup. You may need a blood count to see if you have iron-deficiency anemia.

• You should have your menstrual periods at the normal time. If there's a delay of two weeks or more, see your doctor.

• If at any time you can't see or feel the IUD string, *but you have no other symptoms,* wait for your next period to see if the string comes down. Use an alternate contraceptive method on the possibility that the IUD has fallen out.

• If the IUD does fall out, see your doctor or clinic promptly.

• If your partner complains that the IUD string is irritating, you can ask your doctor to trim it shorter.

• Trouble signals connected with IUDs are fever, chills, pain and vaginal discharge. Get medical attention right away if you have any of these symptoms.

• Statistically, IUD users have somewhat higher rates of pelvic inflammatory disease (p.i.d. usually affects the Fallopian-tube and ovary system), as well as higher rates of ectopic pregnancy. It is particularly important for you to have prompt medical attention if you have an overdue period or any signs of infection such as pain or fever.

It is estimated that more than 50 million women throughout the world take oral contraceptives. In recent years, concern about health risks and side effects from pill use has caused many women to stop using them.

"The pill" is still the choice of women under thirty in the United States. But among couples in which the woman is between thirty and forty-four, voluntary sterilization of either the man or the woman is gaining ground at about the same rate pill use is decreasing—amounting to about 30 percent of the couples in this age group.

The two basic types of oral contraceptives are the combination pill, containing the steroidal female sex hormones estrogen and progesterone, and the progesterone-only pill, sometimes called the mini-pill. The combination pill prevents the ovaries from releasing eggs; the mini-pill interferes with either fertilization or implantation of the egg.

Oral contraceptives can be obtained only by prescription in the United States. Your doctor will probably take a rather detailed medical history and give you a thorough examination. The pill is usually not prescribed for women who have had a stroke or other blood-vessel problem, liver disease, unexplained vaginal bleeding, cancer of the breast or uterus, or who might be pregnant. Some conditions may become worse with oral-contraceptive use. Among them are migraine headaches, depression, asthma, fibroid tumors, heart or kidney disease, high blood pressure, diabetes and epilepsy.

Smoking greatly increases the pill user's risk of a heart attack, stroke and blood clots in the veins. Young women with no risk factors other than smoking may still choose the pill, but should be prepared to switch methods as they become older.

Health risks associated with the pill have been found to increase with long use and with age; current medical advice is to switch to another birth-control method when you reach your late thirties or have been on the pill for several years.

There's no evidence at this time that oral contraceptives increase the risk of cancer. The pill has been found to reduce the incidence of benign breast lumps that may be the forerunners of cancer, though breast cancer already started may be stimulated by the estrogen in oral contraceptives. The pill also appears to protect, to some degree, against genital herpesvirus and rheumatoid arthritis. Dysmenorrhea, or menstrual cramps, almost always becomes milder or clears up when a woman takes oral contraceptives.

The combination oral contraceptive is the most effective reversible birth-control method known. (If it is stopped, the woman usually becomes fertile again.) Surgical sterilization, on the other hand, is not reversible and is completely effective in preventing pregnancy.

When the pill fails to protect, it's usually because the woman forgot to take a pill or two. If you miss taking one pill, take it the following morning, or just as soon as you realize the omission. Risk of pregnancy is quite low with only one or two skipped pills. But if you fail to take your pills for more than two days, call your doctor for advice on how to resume. Meanwhile, use another contraceptive method.

Side effects of oral contraceptives vary widely. Many women have none at all. In others, discomfort and symptoms may be only temporary and disappear after two or three months. In some, the side effects are so severe that the pill must be discontinued.

What effects? That depends on your own body's response to hormone dosage. Most combination pills—those with estrogens and progestogens—will suppress your own estrogen production. The pill, even though doing its intended job of preventing ovulation, could cause symptoms associated with too much estrogen, too little estrogen, too much or too little progestogens. Too much estrogen can lead to bloating, weight gain, headaches, nausea and vomiting —very much like early pregnancy symptoms. Too little estrogen may produce dry, shrunken vaginal tissues and breakthrough bleeding, very much like the estrogen deficiency of menopause. Oral contraceptives containing low amounts of estrogen can produce spotting or complete lack of menstrual flow. Estrogen may clear up acne if you had it before starting the pill. Progestogens may set off skin eruptions you didn't have before.

This explains why your physician may need to adjust your oral-contraceptive dosage or switch to a different formulation during the months after you start the pill.

For women who can use it comfortably, the pill has real advantages. It causes no inconvenience at the time of intercourse, permitting the spontaneity that may be particularly valued. It is almost completely effective—provided it's used properly. In most women the pill produces light menstrual periods with no cramping. Women who have endometriosis are sometimes relieved by oral contraceptives.

If you like the convenience and dependability of oral contraceptives, here are a few points that may help make it work for you:

• When you first go on the pill, have a backup method, such as diaphragm, condoms or foam at hand.

• Look ahead at your supply of pills and the number of times your prescription can be refilled. Make an appointment with your physician *before* you come to the end of your supply.

• If you run into serious problems, such as bad headaches or leg pains, call your doctor immediately.

• If you use the services of a clinic, ask for a phone number to call if you have questions.

• When you want to go off the pill and become pregnant, use an alternate birth-control method for three to four months after stopping the pill to be certain there will be no harmful effects on your baby when you conceive.

• Use supplementary vitamins and minerals during the time you're on the pill, because oral contraceptives increase some nutritional demands, especially for vitamin B_6 and folates. Prenatal multivitamins are good for this purpose.

Sterilization: Consider It Permanent

If you're really certain you do not want to become pregnant, no matter what the future holds, you'll probably consider sterilization by surgery. This is the world's leading contraceptive method as the present decade opens. At last count, more than 7.5 million married couples in the United States had either one or the other partner surgically sterilized.

For women there are several kinds of surgical procedures to achieve sterility. Hysterectomy—complete removal of the uterus and cervix, and sometimes also the tubes and ovaries—will of course cause sterility. It has become fairly common in the United States for women to have this operation for purposes of contraception. But it's a major operation, it has effects on the whole body, and these days it's not generally recommended as a contraceptive measure unless there are strong health reasons such as excessive bleeding and irregularity, or precancerous condition of the tissues.

The predominant female sterilization operation is the tubal ligation, which literally means tying off the Fallopian tubes. Actually, the word "ligation" is used to describe any of several approaches—cutting, clamping, plugging, cauterizing and freezing, to name some. Any of these approaches can be employed; whatever is effective in blocking the pathway by which the egg moves from ovary to uterus.

Tubal ligation leaves the female system intact. It does not stop ovulation or menstruation, but the eggs produced by the ovaries can't move through the tubes to be fertilized and are disposed of by body tissues. Nor can the sperm swim up the tubes to fertilize an egg.

Whatever the means, interfering with the egg-sperm traffic inside the Fallopian tubes is highly effective in preventing conception. The very rare failure may be due to a process called recanalization. In such instances, the tissue forms a new channel, and the egg (or the sperm) can find its way across the gap in the tube. A similar phenomenon has been observed after interruption of the male vas deferens tube, but again, it occurs so infrequently that it is not a practical consideration.

Probably more important to you than the particular way your tubes are blocked or severed is the type of operation you have. From the 1880s into the first quarter of this century, most tubal ligations were carried out in connection with childbirth. Today the operation may be performed at any time. Complications are, in fact, less likely when it's done at some time other than immediately after childbirth. But it may be more convenient for you as an individual, and save an extra hospitalization, to have ligation done just after the birth of a child.

The three main surgical approaches to the tubes are the standard laparotomy (literally, cutting into the flank, which here means the abdominal wall), and two recent techniques known as Band-Aid laparoscopy and mini-laparotomy (or mini-lap).

In standard laparotomy, the abdominal incision is made in such a way as to permit the surgeon to cut and tie the tubes as they lie in place. In laparoscopy, the surgeon works inside the abdomen, using a lighted surgical telescope. In mini-laparotomy, the tubes are literally fished out through a very small incision.

INSIDE JOB: BAND-AID LAPAROSCOPY

In the Band-Aid procedure, either one or two small incisions are made in the abdomen. These openings are only about one-fourth to one-half inch in length. When the viewing instrument, or laparoscope, is coupled with the operating instruments, only one incision is needed; when the instruments are to be manipulated separately, two incisions are made. Carbon-dioxide gas—the familiar gas we exhale and that forms the bubbles in seltzer—is carefully pumped into the abdominal cavity to form a kind of viewing chamber so the surgeon can locate the Fallopian tubes. With the laparoscope, the operator performs the surgery from the outside looking in. The tubes may be interrupted by electrocautery, scarring the tubes closed, or by applying clips or rings that block the passage. The operation may involve an overnight hospital stay, or it may be an outpatient procedure in which you walk out after a few hours—but you'll need someone to help you get home.

MINI-LAP: THE EXTERIOR APPROACH

Mini-laparotomy involves a small incision—only an inch or a bit more—in the abdomen. First, a slim surgical tool placed in the uterus through the vagina is manipulated to bring the closed end of the uterus, or fundus, up against the abdominal wall, where the surgeon can see it as a small bump. This is a guide to making the incision exactly where both tubes will be directly beneath the opening. The surgeon lifts out each tube in turn and carries out the clipping and tying. The incision is closed and stitched. Complica-

STERILIZATION

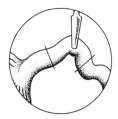 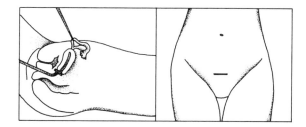

Mini-lap. *Tube shown* (left) *held by clamp. Marked section may be removed or closed off with clips or rings. Instrument in uterus* (center) *positions tubes to be "fished" through opening. Incision* (right) *is just above pubic hairline.*

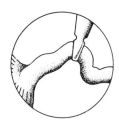 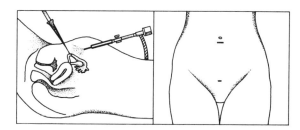

Tubal ligation by laparoscopy. *Tube may be grasped* (left) *by cautery device and closed by burning, or may be pulled through ring, or closed with clips. Procedure is done inside the abdomen* (center), *which is inflated with carbon-dioxide gas to permit viewing by lighted instrument inserted through second incision, just below navel. The two incisions* (right) *are very small, "Band-Aid" size.*

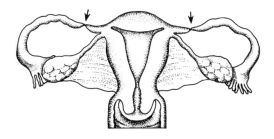

After tubal ligation, Fallopian tubes are closed (arrows). In other methods, severed ends of tubes may be more widely separated or tucked into uterine tissues or have loops or cauterized ends.

tions are infrequent and readily managed when they occur, according to obstetrical surgeons who prefer the minilap. Recovery, they add, is rapid. Ordinary activity can be resumed in a relatively short time. The best candidate for the mini-lap is a nonobese woman with a uterus that can be moved readily. Earlier operations, adhesions from infections, tumors or endometriosis may make the mini-lap impracticable.

THE VAGINAL ROUTE: COLPOTOMY

The Fallopian tubes can also be reached through the vagina, in an operation that leaves no scars on the abdomen. The incision is instead made through the vaginal tissue ("colpotomy" comes from the Greek word for vagina, *kolpos*). When the tubes are exposed through this opening, one of the standard ligation methods—cutting, tying, clipping or blocking—is used. When this procedure is done with the aid of a viewing instrument, the endoscope, the method is called culdoscopy (visual examination of the vagina). In the experienced hands of surgeons trained in this procedure it is as safe and satisfactory as laparoscopy.

MALE STERILIZATION: VASECTOMY

Millions of men have undergone sterilization by surgical severing of the two slim tubes—the vasa deferentia—that lie along the testicles. When the "vas" tubes are interrupted, sperm no longer reach the

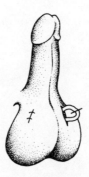

Vasectomy: *Usual bilateral incision site is shown on the left. The vas deferens tube (the tube through which semen flows from the testicle) is shown pulled through small incision on the right. After interruption of the vas, a sperm count is mandatory in a few weeks to make certain that no sperm is getting through the duct.*

ejaculatory duct. The man's sexual function and ejaculate volume are not affected; the only difference is that the seminal fluid cannot impregnate a woman. The operation is usually done by a urologist, and as commonly performed today it is safer, simpler and cheaper than tubal ligation of the woman. Surgical complications are rare. Occasionally a hematoma (collection of blood) in the scrotal tissues or infection may occur. These can be taken care of by the urologist.

The vasectomy is performed under local anesthesia. Incisions are two half-inch openings through which the tubes are located, drawn out and cut or blocked. The man usually is able to resume activity after a day's rest, sexual activity within a few days. Some pain and soreness can persist for one to two weeks.

The most important point to keep in mind about a vasectomy is that the man is not immediately sterile following the operation. Alternate means of contraception should be used until six to ten ejaculations later and until a sperm check by the doctor provides the "all clear" signal.

IF YOU CHANGE YOUR MIND

Surgical sterilization of either the male or the female is virtually fully effective. In the rare cases where pregnancy has occurred after tubal ligation or vasectomy, the tissues may have re-established the interrupted channel. In men, live sperm may survive in the tubes longer than expected. In very rare cases the man possesses a third vas deferens tube that wasn't discovered at the time of surgery.

Can the tubes in either male or female be rejoined if the owner has a change of heart and wishes to be fertile again? It is surgically possible, and has been carried out many times, to achieve reanastomosis, which means that the open ends of the tube are sewn together so the channel becomes patent, and the passage is clear once more. But this microsurgery doesn't necessarily restore fertility.

Candidates for sterilization are best advised to consider it permanent. A few top specialists in sterilization reversal have achieved success in as many as 40 to 60 percent of patients seeking restoration of fertility. But for women, there's a considerable risk of ectopic pregnancy because of damaged tubes. If you should ever need a sterilization reversal, it's best to consult a surgeon who is experienced in this field.

If you're thinking of sterilization surgery, consider the following:

• Talk it over with everyone involved—your doctor, your partner. Ask yourself the hard questions: If your children died, if you divorced, if you remarried—might you regret being sterilized or wish to bear another child? Would realization of your loss of fertility cause emotional upset?

• Is your physician comfortable with the procedure? Some doctors will agree to sterilize only women who have had children. Has the doctor chosen the surgical method to be used and described it fully to you? Have you and your doctor discussed different sterilization procedures?

• Check your insurance or health-care coverage to see if it covers sterilization surgery.

• Is there a waiting period before your surgery can be scheduled? Are a spouse's consent and signature required?

Abortion: Medical Termination of Pregnancy

Ending an unwanted pregnancy by expelling the fetus, a topic of passionate debate today, is nonetheless one of the options in birth control. More than a million legal abortions were performed in the United States during the last recorded year—a rate of almost one abortion for every three live births. But even these statistics can't match those of nature herself. Possibly 40 percent of all conceptions are aborted spontaneously, as if to deny maturation and birth to a defective fetus.

During almost three quarters of the present century, medically induced abortion was prohibited on moral grounds. But long before, doctors had been forbidden to perform abortions for other reasons. In presanitation times, any surgery at all was terribly dangerous, and the risk of maternal death was considered too great to take.

Going back to the thirteenth century, the existence of the fetus was not even recognized in English law until it reached the stage of "quickening" or making perceptible moves inside the womb, about the fifth month of pregnancy. This meant that where abortion was illegal or criminal, the law could apply only to pregnancies past the stage of quickening; there was no other way actual pregnancy could be proved.

The quickening doctrine, we are told by historian James C. Mohr in his book *Abortion in America,* was still in effect both in England and the United States in the early nineteenth century. Women were legally free to terminate a condition that *might* turn out to be pregnancy right up to the time fetal movement occurred and confirmed the pregnant state. After that, purposely expelling it was considered abortion.

Even so, interrupting a pregnancy before the fifth month was traditionally written and spoken about in heavily veiled terms, as treatment for "suppression" or "blockage" of the menses. In common talk and in some books, getting pregnant might be referred to as "taking a cold." And strangely enough, the medicines prescribed for these conditions of "female weakness" were precisely those used knowingly to produce abortion. They included heavy purges, accompanied sometimes by bleeding, hot sitz baths, douches with fairly powerful drugs, and injections into the uterus.

Professor Mohr reproduced in his book some newspaper advertisements by abortionists in Boston about mid-nineteenth century. Both doctor and woman patient carried on the fiction that the lady's complaint was "irregularity," which if neglected would cause "innumerable frightful effects which sooner or later terminate in incurable consumption."

In a not so subtle hint about the real purpose of the "irregularity" medicines, advertisements included warnings like this, for French Periodical Pills: "The only precaution necessary to be observed is ladies married should not take them as they are sure to produce a miscarriage almost without the knowledge of the patient, so gentle yet active are they."

And for the same pills, a recommendation that seems to bear a sly double meaning: "Have been used by females embracing the gentility and most of the nobility of France, for the last 23 years."

The pills and potions intended to induce abortion were rarely medically effective, any more than a punishing laxative would be. They may occasionally have triggered an abortion in a woman inclined to miscarry anyway. But abortionists were prepared with other methods when the pills failed; many of them performed surgi-

cal abortions. Home medical-advice books also recommended strenuous exercise, especially horseback riding. And some practitioners
would resort to extracting a tooth, in hope that shock and pain
would succeed in bringing on the missing menses.

In 1973 a Supreme Court decision made a woman's right to abortion the law of the land. The Court's decision did not settle the
political, moral and religious issues of abortion; indeed, it brought
the subject into great prominence through vociferous public debate.
At the same time, legalization has had profound effects on public
health. Illegal abortions were almost completely replaced by legal
procedures under competent medical supervision, with the resulting
abrupt drop in complications, disability and death. Before the
Court's decision, about a hundred American women were reported
dead each year of complications from illegal abortions. Since then,
the annual reported death toll is five or six. Each year the rate of
complications and severe illness from abortions gets lower and
lower. Much of this improvement is also due to the fact that more
women are getting their abortions earlier in the course of pregnancy, and abortions done before twelve weeks' gestation are generally simple, with a speedy recovery.

The number of abortions per year is still increasing in the United
States, but the rate of increase is slowing down. A primary reason
for the increase may be that more and more women are departing
from the pill and the IUD. The barrier methods of contraception,
with their freedom from complications and side effects, nevertheless
have higher failure rates; and women have opted in many cases to
use these methods with abortion as a backup if it's needed. Thus,
unplanned pregnancies can be the result of:

1. Unprotected sexual intercourse due to ignorance or lack of
   motivation to use contraceptives
2. Use of a method, but failure in practice

If you find yourself with an unwanted pregnancy, only you can
decide what to do. Though the decision is a lonely one, a great deal
of information, support, guidance and reassurance is available to you
today. For example, you should know that the type of procedure,

the health risks, and the pain and discomfort involved in abortion depend primarily on the stage of gestation.

For a very early abortion, a *mini-suction* procedure can be performed in the doctor's office. This consists of a gentle vacuuming of the lining of the uterus with a soft plastic tube. This procedure causes the lining to slough off, just as it does normally during a menstrual period. For this reason it is also called *menstrual extraction*. It is performed as soon as a pregnancy is suspected, sometimes when a period is due but not yet overdue. This can overcome some scruples, since it has not been established that there is a pregnancy, and will not be until the doctor examines the tissue removed. Some studies have found that as many as 30 percent of mini-suction "abortions" were done on women who actually were not pregnant.

Early abortion (EA), performed in the first trimester between the seventh and twelfth week of pregnancy, is another type of vacuum procedure. It will probably be performed with a larger tube, or cannula, and may be followed by curettage, a procedure in which the doctor goes over the uterine lining with a spoonlike surgical instrument, the curette. The whole process takes only ten minutes or so. It is relatively painless, but there's likely to be some discomfort and cramping.

Surgical curettage, a procedure in which instruments are used to scrape the endometrium, or uterine lining, may be carried out at any stage of pregnancy up to the twenty-fourth week. The two approaches are the *dilation and curettage* (D&C) usually used up to the twelfth week, and *the dilation and evacuation* (D&E), for abortions from the thirteenth week.

The D&C is done under anesthesia and may be done on an "in-and-out" basis, in which you go home the same day, or it may call for an overnight hospital stay. In this procedure the cervix is first dilated by instruments, and then the curette is used. Suction equipment may also be used to remove the uterine contents.

In the D&E, the cervix is dilated as in the D&C; but because the uterus is now so enlarged, mechanically forcing the mouth of the cervix to open wide enough can cause difficulty. Some surgeons insert laminaria tents on the day before the operation. These are small sterilized sticks of seaweed material that absorb fluid and swell up gradually, causing the cervix to dilate gently and painlessly.

During the operation the surgeon uses instruments to evacuate the uterus.

Another surgical procedure used in late abortions—usually when other methods are not medically advisable or when sterilization is to be done at the same time—is *hysterotomy* (not to be confused with hysterectomy, which is removal of the uterus). Through an abdominal incision, the uterus wall is opened and the contents are removed with instruments. The uterus is left intact, but scar tissue will form. If future pregnancies are planned, they will probably need a Caesarean delivery.

Nonsurgical late abortion is performed by *instillation*. In this procedure a special fluid is injected into the amniotic sac to bring on labor contractions and delivery of the fetus and placenta, as in childbirth. Saline, or salt solution, is one fluid used; the other is a solution containing prostaglandin, a body chemical that affects muscles and blood vessels.

Instillation abortion can be done only after the sixteenth week, so if you were twelve weeks pregnant and considering this procedure, you would be asked to wait about a month until the fetus can be expelled by induced labor.

The steps of instillation abortion are as follows: First, a thorough examination is undertaken with particular attention to kidney function if a saline abortion is planned. Then blood and urine tests are administered, as well as a check for Rh factor (if it is negative, you should get a RhoGAM® injection (immune globulin) after the abortion to protect future children from the "blue baby" syndrome (insufficient oxygen in the blood). After a local anesthetic in the skin, a hypodermic needle is inserted into the uterus through the abdominal wall. Amniotic fluid is withdrawn and replaced with the solution through the same syringe.

Afterward you wait for contractions to begin. This can happen within a few hours or it may take a couple of days. You may feel cramps or nausea. When labor starts—like heavy cramps to anyone who hasn't experienced it before—the process is simply the same as giving birth, except that an incomplete fetus will be expelled.

More recently, vaginal suppositories containing prostraglandin have become available to induce abortion between twelve and twenty weeks gestation or for use after an intrauterine fetal death.

Obviously, the later the abortion is performed the more physical strain it involves. You may feel tired or weak, particularly if you've had some blood loss, but earlier fears that women would suffer severe depression following abortion have not been borne out. For the most part, the patient generally feels relieved.

It's wise to get information and counseling before you make a firm decision on abortion. Planned Parenthood offers professional, nonjudgmental guidance; the agency has offices or clinics in almost every major city. (If you're in a smaller city or town, the information operator in the nearest large city can give you Planned Parenthood's number there. Then a toll call can get you an abortion counselor.) Another source is your local health department, which can supply the name of a clinic or abortion service that meets acceptable health standards.

Free-standing abortion clinics vary widely in the quality of their services and in the cost. They will be medically supervised, but the doctors are not necessarily trained in gynecology. To select the best and safest abortion service, you might:

• Get a recommendation from a physician you trust.
• Consult a hospital's emergency room staff or gynecology clinic, who probably know which abortion clinics are the best ones.
• Ask the local Planned Parenthood chapter. This agency does not operate abortion clinics, but can direct you to them.

No responsible agency or counselor will ever urge you to have an abortion. Some agencies are committed to urge you not to have an abortion, and will offer prenatal care, assistance in childbirth, and help in caring for the child or placing it for adoption. In any case, the decision must be your own.

Generally speaking, you would be wise to avoid advertised hotline numbers in newspapers and offers of free pregnancy tests connected with commercial abortion clinics (these clinics may perform "abortions" on women who are not pregnant). You can get a pregnancy test from Planned Parenthood, without pressure to have, or not have, an abortion. Avoid places that have an obvious commercial interest in doing abortions.

New Ideas: Contraceptives You Might Buy Tomorrow

Medical research has a dazzling array of new contraceptives waiting in the wings, being developed, being tested, or being readied for approval by the Food and Drug Administration, which requires scientific proof of safety and effectiveness. While these preparations are going on, only a marketing soothsayer could tell which new products will be most effective, most convenient to use, most tuned in to lifestyles of the people who will choose them. As this is written, here are some samples of new, not yet available contraceptives.

Among inert barrier-type devices. Collagen—an organic protein like that in our own bones, tendons and cartilage—is puffed into a supersoft sponge that is simply poked into the vagina, where it clings in place, covering the cervix. It captures and absorbs the male ejaculate and helps maintain the natural acid environment of the vagina. It can be removed after a suitable period following intercourse, washed and reinserted.

Custom-fitted cervical caps of soft plastic made for the individual woman are being researched at the University of Chicago. The physician makes an impression of the cervix, using the same nontoxic material used by dentists for tooth impressions and by eye specialists for contact-lens impressions. The finished cap has a one-way valve that lets menstrual flow and uterine mucus out, and keeps semen from getting in.

Regular cervical caps, at this writing not yet available in the United States, are widely used in Europe.

Among chemical contraceptive methods. Hormone research in contraception is developing fast, as scientists learn more about the biochemistry of the human body. The familiar female sex hormones, estrogen and progesterone, are being tested in new application forms, aimed either at blocking ovulation or preventing implantation without triggering side effects or causing complications.

One method for aiming the dosage right at the target instead of the whole body is a hormone-releasing vaginal ring made of flexible plastic. Placed in the vagina by the user, it emits a low and continuous dose of hormones. It is believed this system will prevent the most-feared risks of the pill: heart attacks, strokes and blood clots. The user removes the ring about every three weeks to interrupt the continuous effects of hormones, waits a few days to allow shedding of the endometrium, and inserts it again. Hormones have also been given in skin-implant pellets, where they provide continuous low dosage for up to a year.

A special class of naturally produced hormone substances, peptides, are involved in the reproductive cycles of both men and women. Research scientists in Finland, for example, have reported a simple nasal spray containing LRH (for luteinizing hormone-releasing hormone) was highly effective in stopping ovulation and therefore preventing conception. Women test subjects said it was pleasant and easy to use.

The possibilities of ill effects from long use of steroidal sex hormones in oral contraceptives have concerned medical science for years. Researchers are now exploring various peptides, for contraception that doesn't add a steroid burden to the body, as well as for male contraception in new forms, such as nasal sprays.

Prostaglandins, the same substances used in instillation abortions, have long been known for their powerful effects on contractile muscles and for their ability to induce abortion. Gynecologic researchers are continuing to look for ways to apply prostaglandins to induce menstruation on a regular basis—an approach that would eliminate the fertilized egg if conception had taken place by bringing on very early abortion without the need to know whether pregnancy has started. Among the methods of prostaglandin application being studied: medicated tampons, slow-release vaginal suppositories, plastic devices to release prostaglandin inside the vagina.

PROFILES OF CONTRACEPTIVE "IDEALS"— WHAT THEY USE

The diaphragm
1. The user is a young married woman who wants to space her children. She and her husband are highly motivated, so she is not likely to forget or neglect to insert the diaphragm; nor would it bother either of them to disrupt a magic moment in order to put it in after love-making has started. If at any time the diaphragm fails, they are in a position either to have an early abortion or to carry the pregnancy to term.
2. Another user is a college girl or career woman who is very comfortable with her body, responsible and consistent in using her diaphragm. She has a stable sex relationship with a man. In case of contraceptive failure she is willing to have an abortion or continue a pregnancy.
3. A third type of candidate is a woman who smokes, who has high blood pressure, a heart or liver condition, or another medical problem making it inadvisable to use the pill, or who cannot use the IUD because of bleeding or cramps. She too is willing to use abortion in case conception occurs or to carry a pregnancy if it would not endanger her own health.
Condom, foam, cream and jelly
1. The user doesn't have sexual intercourse very often, but wants to be prepared for unexpected opportunities. She uses spermicides according to directions and sees that her partner uses the condom correctly. She keeps careful track of her menstrual cycles, and is ready to deal with an unwanted pregnancy.
2. Another user is a young person just becoming sexually active who is unwilling to consult the family doctor for contraceptive advice, or who does not have ready access to a clinic. Here it's doubly important to be consistent and thorough in using the nonprescription methods and to keep a careful record of menstrual cycles, like user Number 1.
Oral contraceptives
1. The user doesn't smoke. She has no medical problems such as liver or circulatory disease. No significant incidence of strokes, heart attacks, or clotting disorders has occurred in her immediate family.
She is still under thirty-five, and her habits are regular, so she's not likely to skip taking a pill. It's important to her to

avoid all possibility of pregnancy—she may be strongly opposed to abortion—so she wants the almost 100 percent effectiveness the pill offers when it's used exactly as directed.

2. She may be a very young girl who needs highly effective contraception and doesn't have ready access to abortion.

The intrauterine device

The user wants a contraceptive that works all the time, without the risk of forgetting a pill or the nuisance of preparing for intercourse with foam, diaphragm or condom. She knows that with these other methods she might slip up and have unprotected intercourse. She has never had gonorrhea, pelvic infection or an ectopic pregnancy. She is not anemic and her menstrual periods are normal, without excessive bleeding or cramps.

Tubal ligation

1 The candidate for sterilization lives in a stable sex relationship and is positive she will never wish to bear any or more children. She has thought seriously of her possible situation if (a) her children were killed, or (b) she was widowed or divorced, and wished to marry a man who wanted children.

2 Another candidate is a woman who has a physical or medical condition in which either childbirth or abortion might be dangerous for her.

Vasectomy

The male candidate for sterilization is a man who is mature and extremely confident of his masculinity. He too is able to consider the questions of loss of existing children or any future marital changes in which more children could be wanted; and even in light of these possibilities he is certain that he wants to become permanently sterile.*

Be sure you are able to make a free and informed decision about the contraceptive method best for you, remembering that a health-care provider or self-help clinic may have a bias favoring or opposing certain methods. Any method that is medically safe for you should be open for your consideration.

*A confirmed bachelor had a vasectomy—because, he said, he didn't want to risk being named in any paternity suits!

8

INFERTILITY: PROBLEMS IN ACHIEVING THE WISHED-FOR CONCEPTION

While millions of people go to considerable trouble to prevent pregnancy, a great many others—estimated at 3 1/2 million persons, or 10 to 15 percent of all married couples—are unwillingly childless. For many, the emotional burden of failure to conceive, or of repeated spontaneous abortions, amounts to personal tragedy.

In recent times, however, remarkable advances have been made in detecting causes of infertility, and in ever increasing numbers, in reversing these conditions and enabling the childless to become parents. Today more than half of the couples with fertility problems can be helped.

But first you must determine if there is a problem. Infertility experts generally define the condition as failure to conceive after one year of unprotected sexual intercourse at a rate of about twice a week. About 85 percent of couples trying to have a baby will achieve pregnancy within a year; the remaining 15 percent may need medical help. But a woman who is past thirty when she starts trying to conceive should probably see her doctor when six months pass without a pregnancy; there's less time to lose if a problem is present.

Female Factors in Infertility

Throughout most of history, barrenness was considered a condition of women only; in patriarchal societies the failure to bear sons was also attributed to some shortcoming of the woman (a fault nearly as bad as barrenness; today we know, of course, that it is the male's chromosomes that determine the sex.)

Blocked or damaged Fallopian tubes are a predominant cause of infertility in women. Defects in cervix or uterus, often surgically correctible, are another cause either of failure to conceive or of repeated spontaneous abortions. Cystic ovaries, called Stein-Leventhal syndrome, are treated medically or surgically. Endometriosis— the disease of displaced uterine tissue—produces scars and adhesions that may lead to sterility. Hormone deficits from any of a number of causes can lead to ovulation failure. In a small proportion of infertility cases, the woman has antibodies that attack and disable sperm; her body's natural defense system for warding off viruses and bacteria has taken exception to the male sperm as well. Some men also develop antibodies that destroy their own sperm.

Besides problems of the reproductive tract itself, a woman may be infertile because of diseases such as diabetes or thyroid disorder, emotional stress, extreme overweight or underweight, and other problems of general health. In some, failure to conceive may be a matter of badly timed or infrequent intercourse, an intact hymen, or inadequate penetration of the penis into the vagina. And there are still a few people consulting doctors about their childlessness whose marriages have actually never been consummated in sexual intercourse.

Male Factors in Infertility

Problems in producing sperm account for a good share of male infertility. An infertile man produces either not enough sperm, defective sperm or sperm with inadequate activity—for sperm are supposed to dash about vigorously, lashing their tails, for hours after their release.

Besides the quality and quantity of living sperm, the man's transport system—the set of tubes carrying semen from its source in the testicles to its discharge from the penis—obviously has to be in working order and unobstructed at any point.

As with women, some conditions outside the reproductive tract can affect male fertility. Thyroid or other gland disorders, past infections and excessive use of alcohol are a few of them. In some men, temporary infertility is caused by too high temperatures around the testicles. The human testicles are carried outside the body in the scrotal sac because internal body temperatures are too high for sperm to survive. Occupations that subject a man to excessive heat, such as trucking where the driver's seat is on top of the heated engine, or even wearing underwear that binds the scrotum closely to the body, can lower the sperm count. Hot tubs and sauna baths also can contribute to impregnation failure.

Having intercourse too often or not often enough may also affect a man's fertility. But unlike women, who may become infertile under emotional stress severe enough to prevent ovulation, men don't have true psychological infertility, according to the University of Chicago's Thomas M. Jones, M.D. Men can become impotent under psychic stress. But as long as a man is capable of sexual intercourse, emotional stress by itself has not been found to affect his fertility.

Let us note here that while most women understand the difference between male fertility and virility, or masculinity, many men feel their manhood is called in question during a medical investigation of the couple's childlessness. This is not the case; while an impotent man, unable to perform the sex act at all, is certainly unlikely to impregnate a woman, the causes of infertility we discuss here occur in couples who enjoy a normal, regular sex life.

Tests and Treatment for Infertile Couples

Your doctor may carry out several measures aimed at detecting causes and correcting infertility. Among these are:

• *Medical history.* Generally, both partners are involved in the infertility examination, though an increasing number of single women are requesting help. The doctor will need detailed information on the woman's menstrual pattern, on any pregnancies or abortions she may have had in the past, on pelvic diseases or infections, and any pelvic surgery. General items of medical history will include childhood diseases, medicines that are taken routinely or frequently, any chronic conditions such as diabetes, use of alcohol and cigarettes, diseases that caused death in near relatives, and any exposure at work to radiation and chemicals. Finally, a sexual history is taken, including not only information about the frequency of intercourse but also considerable detail about sexual habits and techniques. With the exception of menstrual history, male partners are questioned similarly.

• *Physical examination.* Routine examination of the throat, ears, eyes, lung function, heartbeat and blood pressure informs the physician about the patient's general health. For women, a pelvic examination and Pap smear will be done, and probably additional laboratory tests will be ordered. Men will get a thorough examination of the genital organs.

• *Testing.* The woman will most likely be instructed in measuring daily body temperature, called basal body temperature (BBT), before getting up in the mornings. This is done for several monthly cycles to find out when and if she is ovulating. The drop-and-quick-rise in temperature indicates ovulation. The man will be asked to produce a sample of his semen, which will be tested for the number and condition of the sperm.

Family physicians, internists, gynecologists and urologists are qualified to undertake tests and treatment of infertility, or they may conduct initial tests and counseling and later refer you to one of the highly specialized infertility clinics or physicians if further investigation and treatment are needed. Do not assume hopeless infertility (unless an untreatable cause is confirmed) until both you and your spouse have a complete examination. The following are some of the tests that may be offered:

FOR FEMALE INFERTILITY

1. Blood tests of follicle-stimulating hormone (FSH) and luteinizing hormone (LH)
2. Prolactin, estradiol and progesterone testing (a blood test)
3. Venereal-disease testing

4. Rubella (testing for German measles)
5. Mycoplasma and toxoplasmosis tests for fungus infections
6. A test for the presence of antibodies that would attack and kill sperm
7. hCG-beta Sub-Unit (human chorionic gonadatropin)—a hormone test
8. Hysterosalpingogram (an x-ray of the uterus and Fallopian tubes in which an opaque dye is used to outline the interior of the organs and show up any blockages).

FOR MALE INFERTILITY
1. FSH and LH blood tests
2. Testosterone tests (for the male hormone)
3. Prolactin test (a hormone test)
4. Semen analysis: sperm count, activity, malformations
5. Semen mycoplasma test for infection of the semen
6. Sperm antibody tests

Many infertility tests and treatment procedures are costly. It may be wise to ask in advance about fees and costs of medications for a proposed course of treatment and to find out whether any of the procedures are covered by your medical insurance.

Besides the basal body temperature record to chart the drop-and-quick-rise in temperature indicating ovulation, two tests of cervical mucus, the Fern test and the spinnbarket test, also provide evidence of ovulation. In the spinnbarket, wet mucus is checked for viscosity. If it stretches into long threads, ovulation time is near. In the other test, mucus is dried on a slide and viewed through a microscope. Ovulation time is indicated when the mucus forms a fernlike crystal pattern on the slide.

Postcoital testing is important, but it can put a strain on the romance of love-making. About twenty-four to thirty-six hours before ovulation is expected (based on all tests and records for finding out when it is to occur), the couple plans intercourse—and never mind if it has to be at eleven o'clock on a weekday morning because of the ovulation schedule or the doctor's office hours. It is suggested that the woman remain on her back with a pillow beneath her hips for fifteen minutes or so immediately following coitus. She must then report to the doctor's office within two hours (some doctors allow four hours) for an evaluation of the sperm she has retained in the vagina. If they are present in sufficient numbers and are active enough, and if the timing of ovulation is just right, this time—or the same time next cycle—may be the lucky one.

Medical researchers are giving increased attention these days to the possibility of luteal-phase defects as a cause of infertility in women. This means the peak production of luteinizing hormone may be too brief, causing a shortage of progesterone, or it may be out of synchrony with the rest of the ovulatory cycle. Some experts believe this defect is responsible for many formerly unexplainable early abortions. When this cause can be identified, hormone treatment can be given at the proper times to stimulate egg follicle development and the forming of the corpus luteum (the progesterone-producing yellow body).

Disorders of the Fallopian tubes account for about 30 percent of female infertility cases. Tubes may be blocked, kinked or fixed by adhesions. Hydrotubation (forcing fluid through the tube to clear it) may relieve the blockage and avoid the need for surgery. Endometriosis can cause adhesions and scarring, permanently damaging the tubes. The best chances for correcting and restoring function in the impaired reproductive apparatus lie in extremely careful examination and testing by infertility experts and in highly specialized surgical techniques if they are needed.

Excitement seized the world on July 25, 1978, when Louise Brown (erroneously called a test-tube baby) was born of an egg fertilized outside her mother's body, then implanted in the uterus and nourished in the normal, baby-as-usual pattern. The assisted conception, conducted in England by Dr. Patrick Steptoe, eliminated the need for Fallopian tubes, which in Mrs. Brown's case were completely missing. If the procedure proves feasible for other women with tube disorders, and if children produced in this way have no more than the average risk of birth defects, demand for the technique is expected to be great. There are many objections on ethical grounds, among them the theoretical possibility that women might be used to carry out pregnancies with the embryos of other people—modern-day versions of Abraham's wife, Sarah, who sent her maid to bear the child she believed she could never have. As this is written, at least one clinic in the United States is using the Steptoe technique to produce in vitro fertilized pregnancies.

Of the men who seek medical help for infertility, as many as half will be found with sperm deficits caused by a varicocele, which is a varicose vein in the scrotum, nearly always on the left side. Blood that should drain from the testicles into the renal vein gets backed up. As a result of this circulatory problem, sperm counts may be low, sperm may not be active enough, and an increased number of sperm defects, such as misshapen heads, are produced.

A varicocele can be detected by physical examination in a doctor's office. It can be surgically corrected. Alternatives to surgery include clomiphene citrate, a drug also used to stimulate ovulation in women. The drug does not correct the varicocele, but it may increase the man's sperm count and improve fertility. In still other cases the male sex hormone testosterone is used to increase the number and the activity of sperm cells.

Although men who have vasectomy surgery for sterilization are advised at the time to regard the operation as a permanent end to fertility, some men later want their fertility restored. New techniques in microsurgery now make it possible for skilled surgeons to rejoin the vas deferens tubes, and the sperm passage becomes clear in about 60 percent of cases. For various reasons, only about half of the men successfully operated on will later impregnate their mates; but even this success rate is astonishing compared to the scant possibilities only a few years back.

It is now also possible to treat infertility caused by sperm antibodies in either the man or the woman. Immunologic infertility may be treated by immune-suppressing drugs that lower the antibody levels. Another method, still new but showing promise, is to extract the man's semen, remove the antibodies before they disable the sperm and then inseminate the woman artificially on the day of ovulation. This technique, called Sperm Washing Insemination Method, or S.W.I.M., is being studied and conducted at New York Medical College.

Alternatives When Infertility Is Definite

When a woman is fertile and capable of childbearing but her spouse has a sperm count low enough to make pregnancy unlikely, doctors (often a gynecologist-urologist team) may assist conception by artificial insemination, using the husband's semen. At the time the woman is ovulating, semen collected from the husband is placed in the vagina by the physician. How does this differ in effect from natural insemination by sexual intercourse? One answer is that a more concentrated semen can be obtained either by using the first ejaculate, which carries more sperm, or by using a pooled dosage from several ejaculations, which may be collected and preserved by freezing.

Artificial insemination by donor (AID) is the impregnation of the woman with sperm from a male donor who is not her husband. Usually the donor is selected by the physician and is not identified to either the woman or her husband. Ideally the donor is free of genetic defects, in excellent health, and physically similar to the husband.

Sterility of the husband is not the only reason for couples to seek artificial insemination. Some are trying to avoid genetic diseases or defects that could be transmitted by the father. A recent study indicates that up to 10,000 births in the United States each year are results of artificial insemination by donors. A disquieting report was one doctor's statement that he had used the same donor for more than fifty inseminations. This could mean, especially in a small or medium-size community, that a great many half-brothers and half-sisters might meet and marry in the next generation, unaware that they are closely related.

Adoption of a child, a happy solution for countless families, has the double boon of providing a child for parents and providing parents for a child. It is not easy to do, as many prospective adoptive parents know. Higher abortion rates and increased use of contraceptives have reduced the number of babies available for adoption; also, more unmarried mothers are keeping their children rather than giving them up for adoption. Qualifying to receive a child is in many cases an arduous process; and the bureaucratic state of affairs in some localities tends to keep parentless children in the care of paid foster parents, often in a succession of homes, and away from couples who wish to adopt legally and permanently.

For more complete information about infertility and help, you may want to read *The Fertility Handbook,* by Judith Alsofrom Fenton and Aaron S. Lifchez, M.D.

9

THE GYNECOLOGIC INFECTIONS

The female genital tract is warm, dark, moist, rich in glands and blood vessels, and bathed in a number of secretions. Its architecture is intricate and, in some ways, fragile. It is profoundly susceptible to infections. In fact, few women escape having some form of infection, usually causing vaginitis (inflammation and irritation of the vaginal tissues), at some time during their life. Each year about 5 million women develop vaginal symptoms severe enough to send them to a doctor.

The male reproductive tract, equally complex, is vulnerable to infections as well; and the act of sexual intercourse itself permits maximum opportunity for the exchange of infectious organisms.

In addition, the human mouth, throat and rectum provide environments favorable to the growth of infectious organisms; therefore cunnilingus and fellatio (oral sex) and anal intercourse can also transmit infection.

The old term "veneral disease" refers to Venus, goddess of love —who, though she ruled over the arts of love-making, certainly seems to have done little to protect mortals from its graver consequences. Most of us tend to think of venereal disease, or VD, in terms of syphilis or gonorrhea, but there are, in fact, five "reportable" venereal diseases in this country: the two just mentioned, and also chancroid, lymphogranuloma venereum and granuloma inguinale. Diagnosing physicians are required by law to report cases of any of these five to public-health authorities, which will try to locate all the sexual contacts of the VD patients in order to offer them treatment and thus halt the spread of disease.

The trend in medicine today is to abandon the old "venereal" classification for a broader one, sexually transmitted disease (STD), so you will increasingly hear the term STD instead of VD. An STD is often—but not always—transmitted by sexual contact. It can also be transmitted by a mother to her unborn or newborn child, between people in close physical but not sexual contact, and even by transfer from contaminated objects.

There are about twenty conditions recognized as STDs. In this chapter we will discuss genital-tract disease (excepting cancer, which is taken up in Chapter 14), including STDs. First, we will take up the most common vaginitis conditions; then the major venereal infections; and finally a number of other vaginal conditions, most of them not among the STDs.

Most Common Vaginitis Conditions

Vaginitis, a broad term for inflammation and irritation of the vaginal tissues, can really damage one's personal well-being. It can itch or burn, and it often produces a copious, foul-smelling discharge, quite different from the normal vaginal secretions. All in all, it's an assault on the nerves and on one's sense of fastidiousness, and it can have serious repercussions on sex life and marriage. ·

But vaginal discharge is not always caused by an infectious agent. Pregnancy, the use of oral contraceptives, or just the cyclic surge of estrogens preceding the menstrual period can cause heavier-than-usual or abnormal secretions from the vagina. Chemically caused vaginitis may result from repeated and excessive douching or from contact with irritants such as perfumed toilet tissue, perfumed tampons, or vaginal sprays. Atrophic vaginitis is caused by the decreased estrogen production of menopause or oophorectomy (removal of the ovaries). Low estrogen levels cause vaginal tissues to shrink and become thin. (See Chapter 13 for ways to manage this condition.) Atrophic vaginitis may also be found in the nursing mother. Foreign-body vaginitis is most often caused by a retained tampon. Also, little girls with vaginitis may have poked some small object like a bead into this very interesting orifice, just as children poke things into their ears and noses. When the doctor locates and removes the foreign object, the condition usually clears up promptly.

Recently a Texas pediatrics team pointed out that when vaginitis occurs in young girls, doctors may suspect and look for shigella, a bacterium usually associated with epidemics of diarrhea. Trudy V. Murphy, M.D., and John D. Nelson, M.D., of the University of Texas Health Science Center in Dallas, explain that the reason shigella selects young girls for vaginal infection is that before puberty, the vaginal tract does not yet have the protective effects of estrogen and is in a neutral or alkaline state. After menarche, the vagina becomes more acidic and can resist invasion by the shigella organism. A child can have the vaginitis symptoms, often with bleeding, without having the diarrhea of classic shigella infection. Shigella also appears in adults as STD.

TRICHOMONIASIS

Proceeding to the actual infections, let us consider one of the most widespread forms of vaginitis—trichomoniasis, or "trich" for short, caused by *Trichomonas vaginalis*. It affects both men and women and its incidence now approaches 3 million cases each year in the United States. In women, trich infection usually produces a lot of discharge, usually foul-smelling, itchy or burning. In the male, this disease can lurk with no symptoms at all or can cause just a slight burning sensation during urination; it can also spread through the male genital and urinary tracts.

The symptomless trait in males really complicates the battle against trichomoniasis (a fact true of several other STDs, sometimes with the sexes reversed). The effect is that males can be unknowing "carriers" of the disease: they can pass it on to new sexual partners or can reinfect an original partner who has been successfully treated. Moreover, trich infection of exposed males is quite prevalent; about 70 percent of the time, the male partner of a woman with trichomoniasis will be found to have the organism in his urethra.

Obviously, if you should get a trichomonal infection, it's essential for both you and your male partner or partners to be examined and treated in order to prevent "ping pong" reinfection for yourself, to stop any possible spread of the disease, and to protect the man's own health.

The wily trichomonad has been responsible for countless marital crises, with probably a high score of permanent breakups. The scenario goes something like this: A woman sees her physician about a miserable case of vaginitis, which on wet-smear analysis turns out to be trich. She's miserable otherwise, too. Her husband believes she's cheating, and that a new sexual partner has given her the disease. Otherwise why should she suddenly develop these genital symptoms after several years of marriage? He doesn't have any symptoms, so he's certain he didn't give her the infection. Moreover, he hasn't been playing around. And that's that.

The doubting spouse should listen to medical advice on this point. Leonard J. Cibley, M.D., of Boston University School of Medicine, who writes extensively both for doctors and patients, quotes Herman Gardner, M.D., of Texas, that *Trichomonas* can probably stay dormant in the body for twenty years or more, until something triggers it to produce symptoms. This protozoan—literally a tiny, primitive animal—can be harbored not only in the vagina and in the male genital tract, but in the urinary and intestinal tracts of both men and women.

Trichomoniasis can be tricky to identify, can mask as another condition and can occur along with other forms of infection. The classic, "textbook" signs aren't really dependable; the same kind of greenish, foamy, ill-smelling discharge may be caused by some other organism, such as *Hemophilus vaginalis,* also called *Corynebacterium vaginale* (and more recently named Gardneralla, after Dr. Gardner, who first described it). This is important to know because different diseases may require different medical treatment. Therefore, if you've had a trichomoniasis successfully treated, and some weeks or months later the same symptoms recur, it might seem logical to call up your doctor and say, "I've got it again. Will you please phone the pharmacy so I can pick up the prescription?"

The error in this approach is that there's an excellent chance you don't have trich but one of the other conditions that resembles it. You could have contracted another vaginitis separately or you could have had more than one kind of infection in the first place, and the treatment that cleared up the trich infection has allowed the other

organism to emerge. It is fairly common for trich treatment to set
off overgrowth of the yeastlike *Candida* (see page 145). So the only
thing to do is go back to your doctor, who will test to be sure what
manner of creature is producing your vaginitis and will then be able
to prescribe medication specifically for your ailment.

Trich sometimes produces only urinary symptoms. Many physicians are now convinced that a tremendous number of "honeymoon
cystitis" cases (see page 148) are actually caused by undetected trichomoniasis.

The symptoms of trichomoniasis can often be relieved by topical
treatment; that is, by medications applied to the vaginal surfaces by
applicators, suppositories or douches. The problem here is that the
topical products, even if they could kill the organisms on contact,
cannot reach and root out all of them. Dr. Cibley explains why:
"The vagina has hundreds of meters of surface area in tiny accor-
dion folds, and the trichomonad can hide in these crevices. Besides,
the organism is almost surely also harbored in the urinary tract. So
the only way to reach protozoa in all these places is through a
systemic instead of a topical medicine. This means giving a drug by
mouth or by injection so it gets into the bloodstream. The effective
drug for trichomonas is metronidazole."

Metronidazole is fairly strong medicine. It can cause some side
effects such as a metallic taste in the mouth, headache and slight
nausea. It is wise to stay away from liquor during treatment with
metronidazole and for a couple of days afterward, because in all
probability, even a small dose of anything alcoholic would bring on
violent nausea. (A chemical used to treat alcoholics is similar to
metronidazole.)

Metronidazole is remarkably effective—scoring over 90 percent
—in treating trichomoniasis. But it's not effective against all other
forms of vaginitis. Metronidazole should be used only when the
infection is very definitely caused by trichomonads or one of the
other metronidazole-sensitive organisms.

Physicians hesitate to use metronidazole in pregnancy or without
strong reasons due to the few reports that it is carcinogenic in rats
and mice. There is no evidence to date that metronidazole causes
cancer in humans. The standard course of treatment with metronidazole for both men and women lasts seven days. But a new

dosage schedule of one large dose, or a large dose divided in two and taken in a single day, has been used experimentally with reported success. The one-dose treatment clearly has the advantages of shortened side effects, a briefer time one must abstain from liquor, and a greater chance for exposed but symptomless men to agree to treatment.

CANDIDIASIS

The second most common vaginal discharge problem, accounting for about 20 percent of vaginitis occurrences, comes from an organism of the *Candida* family, and is also called monilia, or thrush. Yeastlike (often referred to as a "yeast infection") but not a true fungus, *Candida* can lodge almost anywhere in the body, can cause other forms of illness and is so omnipresent that it seems to wait to strike when body defenses are down: during antibiotic or steroid treatment, during pregnancy or when illness has lowered one's resistance. Diabetics are highly susceptible to candidal infection. You may see the infection identified as *C. albicans,* which is actually the pathogen that causes the infection; it's the same disease, specified by its most active and prominent strain.

Candidal vaginitis can be acquired by sexual contact, but it can also result from self-infection from stools or from contact with contaminated objects. The organism is often present in the mouth and rectum and can even be harbored under fingernails.

The symptoms of candidal vaginitis can be maddening, as its sufferers know. Tissues of the labia and vulva may become red and swollen. Vaginal tissues may bear yellow or white patches or plaques, and may produce an irritating discharge. Itching can be severe, especially at night, and urinating or sexual intercourse usually cause painful burning. Men who get candida infection may have no symptoms, just as in trichomonal infection, or they may have some itching and inflammation of the genitourinary area.

Candidal vaginitis is treated with both oral and topical medications such as nystatin, an antibiotic that works against fungus and funguslike organisms, or clotrimazole and miconazole, which are also antifungal agents. Women who have candidal infection during pregnancy are usually given oral medication to prevent the disease in the baby. Infants exposed to *Candida* during passage through the birth canal can develop serious infection of the mouth (thrush), and may get a diaper rash so severe that it leads to other infections.

It's urgently important to treat male partners of women who have candidal vaginitis, just as it is in trichomonal infections. In uncircumcised men, *Candida* may lurk beneath the foreskin. The organism is also found in the semen of a high percentage of men whose female partners have recurrent candidal vaginitis. Physicians usually prescribe a medicated cream to be applied to the penis before and after intercourse. A doctor may also prescribe a preparation for scrubbing hands and nails, or a special mouthwash.

Good general hygiene may help you avoid candidal infection. A lifelong rule for girls and women is to always use toilet tissue from front to back to avoid contaminating the vagina with traces of stool. Good general health is another factor in warding off candidal infection, since it strikes most often when the body is run-down. Many doctors recommend avoiding airtight-crotch underwear and jeans, and may suggest cotton underwear for women susceptible to candidiasis.

If you have a candidal infection, don't douche except as medically advised. If you douche, avoid reinfection from the douche nozzle by cleaning it thoroughly with soap and water after each use. Remember to urinate promptly after sexual intercourse (to prevent infective material from entering the urinary canal). Also, to keep from adding other irritations to any kind of infectious vaginitis, don't use bubble bath, feminine-hygiene sprays, perfumed or colored toilet paper and perfumed tampons. It may help to wash underwear with real soap, not detergent.

HEMOPHILUS VAGINALIS INFECTION

A few years back, many cases of vaginitis and excessive discharge were medically termed "nonspecific vaginitis," a thoroughly unsatisfactory diagnostic handle. It simply meant that the condition was not trichomoniasis, candidiasis or gonorrhea. Today we know that at least 90 percent of the time the "nonspecific" vaginal infection is caused by one organism, *Hemophilus vaginalis* (pronounced *he-MOFFLE-us*), also known as *Corynebacterium vaginale*.

Usually the major problem in *Hemophilus* infection is copious, foul-smelling vaginal discharge. Itching and burning are mild if they occur at all, and any itching usually means that the infection is accompanied by either *Trichomonas* or *Candida,* or both.

Hemophilus infection is usually treated by antibiotics, and medication for the other vaginitis conditions, if present, may be prescribed at the same time. Most doctors recommend that sexual partners be treated simultaneously.

The most effective treatment so far found for *Hemophilus* vaginitis is metronidazole—the same medication that works with trichomoniasis. But because physicians may be wary of prescribing metronidazole repeatedly to the same patient, they sometimes prescribe an antibiotic first, to see if it clears up the disease. The antibiotics most often used against *Hemophilus* are cephradine and ampicillin.

While some physicians oppose douching at any time, whether or not there's a discharge, others think douching is permissible for women who feel they need it for comfort. If you douche, the word is moderation—overdouching can cause vaginitis by itself by drying and shrinking the vaginal tissues. Trying to handle the itching or discharge of a vaginal infection by frequent douching instead of seeking medical treatment is a very bad idea.

CHLAMYDIAL INFECTIONS

Another longstanding medical puzzler is nongonococcal urethritis, or NGU, so named because its urinary-tract symptoms are not caused by gonorrhea. The condition may cause inflammation throughout the genital tract in women, swollen prostates in men, and urinary-tract discharge and painful voiding in both. Scientific sleuthing has now revealed that about half of all NGU cases are caused by *Chlamydia trachomatis,* a very unconventional bacterium once thought to be a virus. This is also the organism that causes eye disease and a kind of pneumonia in newborn babies and infants.

Chlamydial infection brings with it erosion of the cervix, discharge of pus from the cervical canal, urinary and rectal inflammation, and sterility.

Medical authorities believe chlamydial infection is a major public-health problem, and that it may accompany as much as half of all cases of gonorrhea. The standard gonorrhea treatments with antibiotics do not eradicate a concurrent chlamydial infection; and since the infection is sexually transmitted, it's imperative to treat sex partners simultaneously to prevent overlapping reinfection. Clinical specialists recommend a full 21-day course of tetracycline.

"HONEYMOON CYSTITIS"

Pain or burning that occurs while urinating or during intercourse, with a hot sensation that climbs upward in the urinary canal, can certainly occur at any time, honeymoon or not. It got its nickname because of its prevalence at times of high sexual activity and because the mechanics of intercourse can force infective material to back up into the urinary canal and toward the bladder.

The source of this type of infection is usually bacterial, and a number of organisms may be found when the urine is tested. Your doctor may refer to this problem simply as UTI (urinary-tract infection).

Cystitis is highly treatable, usually with sulfa and antibiotic medications. The bad news is that cystitis can return again and again in some women. Many physicians prescribe preventive medication for patients who suffer three or more bouts of cystitis during a year.

Simple preventive measures can help you avoid urinary-tract infections. Empty the bladder before and promptly after sexual intercourse. During the day, empty the bladder regularly when you get the urge. Studies show that women who have recurrent cystitis invariably have bad urinating habits, putting off emptying the bladder long after the "time to go" signal. According to these studies, infection-prone women are also less likely to void following intercourse.

It is also recommended that you drink generous amounts of water —not just fluids such as coffee, tea or soda, but water. A long, long drink of water after love making should be the rule. Having to rise at night to empty your bladder is certainly preferable to suffering the miseries and damage of cystitis.

Venereal Infections

In the nineteenth century a learned physician who presided over England's Royal College of Medicine declared, in his inaugural address, that he fervently prayed that there would never be a cure for venereal disease—for without the prospect of such punishment, unbridled sexuality and licentiousness would sweep through society. Escaping his notice was the fact that venereal disease killed, blinded, or maimed thousands, principally newborns, quite innocent of the deplored "immorality."

After a doctor has reported a new VD case to the authorities, as he must, a public-health officer communicates with each patient, asking the names of his or her sexual contacts in order to advise them to be examined and treated. Their names do not become public record, nor do health officers reveal them to other individuals. Naturally, it's a process fraught with problems, but it is the duty of public-health workers to protect the privacy of every person concerned and to maintain a disinterested position. It is their job to prevent the spread of disease and to protect the health of people who may not know they're exposed or infected.

GONORRHEA

Gonorrhea is not a disease that happens only to "other people," nor is it confined to the undereducated and underprivileged. It is urgent that all sexual contacts of each person diagnosed to have gonorrhea be examined and treated. If you have the slightest reason to think you may have been exposed to it, you should ask your physician to do a gonorrhea culture. Many doctors do not routinely test for gonorrhea during regular examinations of their private patients.

In contrast to some other sexually transmitted diseases where women have symptoms while their male partners do not, gonorrhea is likely to produce acute symptoms in the male while the woman who transmitted it to him has none. However, the long-range effects of the disease are disastrous for both men and women. It can lead to a crippling form of arthritis and it can severely damage the genital, rectal and urinary tracts in both sexes. It can cause permanent sterility in both. As many as 30 percent of infected women will become sterile after a single episode of gonorrhea; after multiple episodes the sterility rate may be over 90 percent. Furthermore, gonorrhea infections increase the risk of ectopic pregnancies. Transmitted by the mother, gonorrhea can cause eye disease in newborn children, and inflamed vulvas and vaginas in baby girls.

Male symptoms of gonorrhea include painful urination and pus-containing discharge from the urinary tract, with the opening becoming red and swollen. Women who get symptoms have similar ones, with inflamed urinary tract and abdominal pain due to infected Fallopian tubes.

The incidence of gonorrhea has risen to epidemic proportions. The infectious organism that causes it has a trait enabling it to develop resistance to antibiotic treatment. Once there was great hope that penicillin alone would eradicate gonorrhea. But instead of perishing as planned, some strains of *Neisseria gonorrhoeae* adapted themselves by developing an enzyme called penicillinase that actually eats up the antibiotic. However, gonorrhea can be cured. There are four different medical approaches for treatment of uncomplicated cases of gonorrhea. The standard treatment for both men and women at this writing is penicillin G injected into the muscle, along with an oral dose of probenecid. Patients who are allergic to either medication may be given oral tetracycline hydrochloride. Some patients who cannot tolerate tetracycline and may not have penicillin are treated with an injection of spectinomycin. Another drug that may be used for gonorrhea is ampicillin. In cases where the patient has been infected with syphilis along with gonorrhea, the incubating disease will be eradicated by any of the gonorrhea treatments except spectinomycin. Tetracycline treatment will usually eliminate chamydial infection that may be present with gonorrhea.

SYPHILIS, THE OLD ENEMY

The infection lues venerea was named syphilis in about 1530 by the Italian physician Girolamo Fracastoro, who published a poem on "the French disease" featuring as its central character a Greek shepherd named Syphilus, or "friend of swine."

The disease is still with us. About 20,000 cases per year are reported by physicians, but public-health officials think several thousand more cases go unreported. Some authorities believe more than half a million cases of "latent" syphilis go unnoticed.

Untreated, syphilis can take an inexorable course from an early, infectious stage with symptoms to a symptomless but damaging stage, and onward to the tertiary stage of irreparable cardiovascular and nervous-system degeneration. Yet a great many syphilis-infected people simply outgrow, or wear out, the disease—they "experience a biologic cure," according to medical texts.

Syphilis is almost entirely acquired by sexual contact, although it is theoretically possible for laboratory workers handling infectious materials to acquire it accidentally. It may be anywhere from ten to ninety days after the contact that the first signs of infection appear, in the form of a primary lesion, or chancre (pronounced *shanker*). This is a buttonlike sore with a rigid border, and it is usually painless. It usually appears in the genital areas of either men or women, and can go unnoticed if it occurs in the female vaginal tract. It can erupt around the rectum, on the lips, nipples or inside the mouth.

This innocuous little sore will go away by itself, without treatment. But the disease has gone underground. In a few weeks all kinds of lesions may start to appear. Palms and soles break out in sores, hair falls out in patches, lymph nodes become lumpy, blisters appear around the genital and rectal areas and in the mouth. These signs, too, will heal and go away even without treatment. When syphilis goes into the latent stage it is still infectious for about another two years. After that, although the disease is no longer infectious, it can systematically destroy the brain and spinal cord, heart, blood vessels, liver, skin and bones.

If a woman has syphilis and becomes pregnant, or acquires the disease during pregnancy, chances are high for stillbirth or for a severely deformed baby.

Treatment before the eighteenth week of pregnancy prevents infection of the fetus. Even after the fetus has been infected, both mother and unborn baby can be treated successfully up until the third trimester. But if treated very late in pregnancy, the infected fetus may already have irreversible birth defects, even though the syphilis spirochete has been destroyed.

The drugs used to eradicate the syphilis organism are penicillin, erythromycin or tetracycline, as for gonorrhea. But dosage forms differ. The possibility that two or more kinds of infection may be present at the same time presents the physician with some fancy therapeutic footwork to perform. As we have seen with trichomonal infection, medication that destroys the syphilis organism can set free a competing organism that had been held in check. A veritable outburst of symptoms can follow. If you're the patient, you may think the original infection has returned, when in fact it's a whole new ball game. The case with other genital infections is similar;

there's a good possibility for several organisms to exist concurrently. The doctor may treat one of them temporarily with topical medications or sulfa tablets until another disease, such as syphilis, has been ruled out. The message is: Keep every follow-up appointment your doctor sets up.

GENITAL HERPES

Herpes simplex virus, or HSV, can cause pure misery, with itching, burning blisters on the labia and vulva, or anywhere throughout the reproductive tract. There are two kinds: HSV-1, which also causes the common cold sore on the lips, and HSV-2, a closely related kind that was once thought to stay below the waist, while number 1 dwelled only above the waist. The territorial boundary no longer prevails, however, and the difference between the two viruses is largely academic; both behave in much the same manner.

HSV infection has been associated with increased risk of later cervical cancer. It is highly contagious, rated about 90 percent transmissible during sexual contact if either partner has an active blister. The virus can spread to newborn babies during delivery, and the infection can kill, blind or severely disable the baby. When a pregnant woman has active HSV lesions at term, physicians usually perform a Caesarean section to prevent infection of the child.

Genital HSV is believed to be the number-two venereal disease in the United States, second only to gonorrhea. It also appears to be spreading rapidly. By all current standards, it is incurable; once in the body, the virus stays there, although treatment can help clear up the symptoms and some therapy helps to suppress active bouts of the disease.

Although the virus doesn't go away, there are periods of quiescence between attacks when the blisters subside. Specialists think the disease is unlikely to be transmitted at these times. But because HSV sores, or lesions, may be on a nonsensitive area such as the cervix, and may not be seen or felt, there is no assurance that at any given time the virus is nontransmissible.

What can help prevent recurrence of active HSV?

Irritation of vaginal tissues from other causes is a known factor in triggering a genital herpes attack. It's important to clear up any vaginal discharge from a coexisting infection. During intercourse, adequate lubrication can help protect the woman from too much friction; vaginal lubricants that can be bought without a prescription can be helpful. Use of a condom can protect the man from excessive rubbing. If he has active HSV blisters, the condom may reduce or prevent pain during intercourse. And, of course, the condom offers a measure of protection if either person is uninfected.

When ruptured HSV blisters are causing extreme pain, there are a number of steps you can take to get relief. A long soak in a tepid bath helps. The virus blister is rather like a burn; exposure to air can cause painful drying; so medication in ointment form can be soothing. Cold packs—washcloths squeezed lightly in the coldest tap water, not ice—can be applied to the labia and vulva.

Application of zinc sulfate—an old medication long in use for other skin lesions—has shown promise and is at this writing under active investigation. At the University of Arizona, an experimental contraceptive, a collagen sponge, distinctly suppressed HSV activity when it carried a dose of zinc sulfate.

A combination of the sulfa and antibiotic agents sulfamethoxazole and trimethoprim has also been reported effective.

Most recently, 2-deoxy-D-glucose, a relative of the blood-sugar glucose, gave dramatic evidence of actual cure of genital HSV in a test group of thirty-six infected women. At the University of Pennsylvania, Herbert Blough, M.D., directed the use of the drug in a gel or creme form, applied to the virus blisters four times a day for three weeks. Symptoms generally disappeared within twelve hours to three days. About 90 percent of the patients were pronounced cured following the three-week treatment. Recurrence of HSV was either prevented or greatly reduced in other patients.

At this writing, 2-deoxy-D-glucose has not yet been licensed by the Food and Drug Administration for general use by doctors. Data are being examined and research continues in order to make certain that the treatment not only works but is safe.

Success has been reported in treating HSV lesions on lip and mouth tissues by swabbing the affected areas with a dye solution, then exposing them to a special shortwave ultraviolet light. This method has also been proposed for the treatment of genital HSV, but a number of specialists say this treatment increases cancer risks and warn against its use.

Other Vaginal Conditions

The Bartholin's glands, located just inside the vagina, are there to secrete mucus. Sometimes the opening of a gland becomes obstructed and a cyst—a saclike plug—will form. Bartholin's cysts are quite common and are usually benign and painless. If one of them starts growing in size or threatens to become inflamed, your doctor may decide to have it surgically removed; in some cases he will recommend leaving the cyst alone or checking it at intervals to see if it is growing. If it bothers you, the physician may prescribe pain relievers, extra rest, and cold and warm applications for relief of discomfort.

A Bartholin's-gland abscess is different from a cyst. It is an infected, boil-like eruption and it is very painful. You should seek a doctor's help. As with any abscess, the doctor will open, drain and cleanse it.

Skene's glands, ducts which lie near the urethra, can develop cysts too, though these are not nearly as common as Bartholin's cysts. Skene cysts may arise in connection with a genital infection such as gonorrhea, so treatment is concurrent with that for the underlying infection.

Venereal warts, condylomata acuminatum, usually appear as cauliflower-like red and spongy masses scattered over the vulva, the surrounding skin and rectal area, and sometimes down onto the thighs. The warts may also spread into the lower vagina, but very rarely invade the upper vagina or the cervix. Like other warts, they are virus infections and are believed to be almost entirely sexually transmitted. They may affect males as well as females, and may be just as acutely painful or disabling for men as for women. In men, venereal warts appear on the penis and around rectal areas. Because the virus may be harbored beneath the foreskin, circumcision is sometimes performed to prevent recurrence of the warts and reinfection of sexual partners.

If the warty growths are not too extensive, the doctor may apply a wart-removing compound, podophyllum resin. This is done very carefully because the medication could deliver a chemical burn if spread over delicate normal tissues. You should never, repeat *never,* try any home remedy for venereal warts. Your physician may prescribe both oral and topical sulfa drugs, or the condition may require surgery.

Condylomata acuminatum can be greatly aggravated by pregnancy. The physician may treat to relieve symptoms but postpone vigorous treatment such as podophyllin or surgery until after childbirth.

Tips on Dealing with Gynecologic Infections

PERSONAL HYGIENE

Make sure everything that enters the vagina is clean. Avoid self-contamination by careful toilet habits. Tampons are often preferable to exterior pads for menstrual use; they prevent chafing of the vulva and the breakdown of menstrual fluids on exposure to air.

PARTNER HYGIENE

Your sexual partner should be free of lesions (eruptions) on the external genitalia. If uncircumcised, he should have the habit of thoroughly cleansing the foreskin and glans (head) of the penis. For both of you, overall bodily cleanliness is important because infectious organisms can be carried on hands and body surfaces.

WHEN SYMPTOMS ARISE

Be candid with all sexual contacts who may be exposed to—or may be the source of—your infection. Get partners treated. If the infection is one of the reportable VDs, get help from, and cooperate with, health department officers, who, in turn, will do all they can to protect your privacy and confidentiality.

CONFIDENTIALITY FOR TEEN-AGERS

The American Academy of Pediatrics recommends to its physician members that VD examinations and treatment of minors be a confidential and private matter between doctor and patient.

PARTNER ALERT

If your sexual partner or husband, without being very specific about it, suggests that you get a "checkup," don't argue. Go.

A Case History: VAGINITIS

Janis R., twenty-six, a very busy advertising copywriter, hated to take time off for a doctor's appointment. But she hated even more the condition she had recently developed —persistent vaginal itching, along with a foul-smelling discharge that was growing more profuse each day.

Discussion of the problem with women friends produced the following opinions:

1. It was probably gonorrhea.
2. She should douche.
3. She should not douche.
4. It was probably a yeast infection.
5. She might be diabetic.
6. For a similar problem, a friend had taken tetracycline.

When Janis finally did get to the doctor's office, she was first given a pelvic examination. After taking a sample of material from the mouth of the cervix for a culture (preparing the gonococcus organism to grow if any was present in the sample) the doctor prepared a "wet mount" of the vaginal discharge by placing a sample of it on a microscope slide, where it could be examined right away.

The doctor saw *Trichomonas vaginalis.* This explained the vaginal discharge. It required a week of treatment with metronidazole. Both Janis and her sexual partner would have to be treated at the same time for it to be effective; otherwise she would very likely become reinfected. They were advised not to drink any alcohol during the course of treatment, or they might become nauseated.

Treatment was fully effective. The gonorrhea culture was negative, and Janis had no further symptoms that would indicate the presence of additional organisms for other kinds of vaginal infection.

10

GYNECOLOGIC SURGERY

Gynecologic surgery is a relatively young field. Despite some suggestive references to possible Caesarean sections in very early times (as in Macduff's being "from his mother's womb ripp'd untimely" in Shakespeare's *Macbeth*), such early emergency procedures were invariably fatal to the mother or were done to rescue the fetus when the mother had died. The modern era of surgery became possible only after the advent of anesthesia and antisepsis in the late nineteenth century, and surgery only became very safe in the twentieth-century antibiotic era. Surprisingly, female surgery began not with hysterectomy but with ovariectomy (oophorectomy, or the removal of the ovaries) and with procedures for urinary incontinence.

Oophorectomy was hailed as a treatment for "female unruliness." Ben Barker-Benfield describes the indications or conditions justifying removal of the ovaries, used by Dr. Robert Battey, a prominent surgeon, between 1860 and 1890:

"Among the indications were a troublesomeness, eating like a ploughman, masturbation, attempted suicide, erotic tendencies, persecution mania, simple 'cussedness,' and dysmenorrhea. Most apparent in the enormous variety of symptoms doctors took to indicate castration was a strong current of sexual appetitiveness on the part of women."

Because removal of the ovaries was believed to be a cure for most forms of "unruliness," many husbands talked their wives into volunteering for this procedure. Today, of course, oophorectomy is done only for primary diseases affecting the ovaries, such as endometriosis, pelvic inflammatory disease, large cysts, or tumors, or in connection with hysterectomy when necessary.

Shortly before Dr. Battey started to operate on imagined pathology, J. Marion Sims, M.D., a prominent gynecologist, was working on a very real problem—that of incontinence. In 1852 Dr. Sims reported the first successful repair of a vesicovaginal fistula (an opening between bladder and vagina, resulting in uncontrollable leakage of urine through the vagina). He is justifiably credited with creating the modern specialty of gynecologic surgery. On the negative side, he is reported to have used cast-off slave women and other indigents as guinea pigs, often operating experimentally, and unsuccessfully, many times on the same woman. And this was in the days before anesthesia!

Removal of the uterus was first successfully performed in 1853 by Walter Burnham, M.D., of Lowell, Massachusetts. High death rates kept the operation from coming into common use, however, until the twentieth century. Once hysterectomy came to be considered "safe," it was advocated at times as a treatment for backache, "pelvic relaxation," heavy or painful periods, for contraceptive purposes and to "prevent" cancer.

We have come a long way from the days of ovariectomy for "cussedness" and hysterectomy for "backache." Nonetheless, some serious questions have been raised about gynecologic surgery. Dilation and curettage (D&C), tubal ligation and hysterectomy are among the most commonly performed procedures in the United States. In countries with a national health system, such as Great Britain, the incidence, and cost, of such surgery are much lower. In the United States, too, hysterectomy rates are lower under prepaid health plans than under fee-for-service medical care. Those figures are used to assert that fee-for-service doctors are doing too much surgery in order to make more money; but an equally convincing case can be made for nationalized health programs and prepaid health plans doing too *little* surgery in order to save money. Figures on the number of "normal" uteruses, found undiseased after removal, also are of little help for proving claims of unnecessary surgery, because many conditions that legitimately require hysterectomy (such as prolapse, chronic pain or urinary incontinence) occur with the uterus perfectly disease-free.

Let's explore some questions you may want to ask yourself and your physicians when you are faced with the prospect of surgery.

* *What are your symptoms?* Except for early cancers, which may have no symptoms at all, the majority of gynecologic problems requiring surgery do cause symptoms. A woman who has sought medical care time and time again for pelvic pain or bleeding, and who has had a number of treatments that did not work, should not be surprised if a physician suggests surgery. Remember, *early cancers* are an exception and may give no warnings. Cancers are biopsied and clearly diagnosed before a decision concerning surgery can be made.

* *Are alternative treatments available?* Dysfunctional (abnormal) uterine bleeding, for example, may be treated with hormones rather than a D&C or hysterectomy. For cervical dysplasia (abnormal surface tissue), cervical conization (removal of cone-shaped piece of tissue), cryosurgery ("freezing"), laser or cautery may be an alternative to hysterectomy. Some physicians advocate hysterectomy for sterilization, but tubal ligation is a safer, cheaper, easier alternative —provided there is no other disease condition in the uterus. Although many physicians regard hysterectomy with vaginal repair as the favored treatment for urine incontinence, some women may be helped by simple hormone treatment, by treatment of a urinary-tract infection or by vaginal repair alone. You should learn as much as possible about alternatives to surgery. Ask your physician about them.

* *What are your own reasons for wanting or not wanting surgery?* Women have been known to ask for a D&C to "clean me out inside," a hysterectomy to end the inconvenience of periods, a tubal ligation to save a failing marriage, or a breast enlargement to attract men. These women may well end up scraped but no "cleaner," depressed about their womblessness rather than their periods, divorced but now sterile as well, or big-chested and still dateless. If you *want* surgery, consider these questions:

1. Are your expectations realistic? (Such as possible relief from chronic pain rather than a remake of your whole existence.)

2. Are you projecting other problems onto your female organs? (Such as expressing marital stress in dyspareunia (pain during intercourse) or blaming a poor social life on breasts that are too small or too large.

3. If you are seeking sterilization, are you quite sure that you will *never* want to bear more children and not just reacting to current pressures from small children or a dissatisfied husband?

If you do *not* want recommended surgery, consider these questions:

1. Do you doubt the need for surgery? If so, there's good reason to get a second opinion.

2. Is your fear rational? Talking out your fears with a counselor, a medical professional or an understanding friend may help to put them in a proper light.

• *Do you need a "second opinion"?* Lately there has been much commotion about this question. Often, particularly in the case of elective procedures, doctors vary in their opinions about the necessity for surgery. Here are some situations in which seeking another medical opinion may be justified:

—When a surgeon is entirely unknown to you and you would like counsel from your regular physician.

—When there is an ongoing medical controversy about the best treatment, such as radical mastectomy or not in the case of breast cancer, or the treatment of early cervical cancers.

In seeking a physician for a second opinion, look for a specialist in the field, preferably with no connection with the first physician. A doctor at a teaching center or a specialist at an outpatient clinic may be good sources of second opinions.

Following are descriptions of some surgical procedures, the reasons for having the operations and what is involved for you.

Hysterectomy

Since this is one of the most common surgical procedures performed in the United States, the possibility of having one is a prospect that will be faced by many women. First, let us examine the somewhat confusing terminology for the various types of hysterectomy:

• Total abdominal hysterectomy (TAH) is the removal through an abdominal incision of the entire body of the uterus, including the attached cervix. The ovaries are left intact.

When an ovary is also removed it may include the connected Fallopian tube (salpingo-oophorectomy). Removal of uterus, tubes and both ovaries is called "total abdominal hysterectomy and bilateral salpingo-oophorectomy" (TAHBSO). If only the right or left tube and ovary are removed, the procedure is TAHRSO or TAHLSO.

• Vaginal hysterectomy is the removal, as in TAH, of the uterine body and cervix only, through the vagina, not the abdomen. This operation is not performed if the uterus is too large or excessively scarred or if exploration of the abdomen is needed.

• Partial hysterectomy is the removal of only part of the uterus, often the uterine body (or central portion), but not the cervix. This is rarely indicated today because it offers few advantages and several disadvantages over TAH or vaginal hysterectomy. It is occasionally necessary when scar formation, bleeding or operative complications prevent accomplishment of total hysterectomy.

• Radical hysterectomy is often done for uterine cancer. This procedure involves excision of a wide margin of tissue along with the uterus, and removal of associated lymph nodes.

Reasons for hysterectomy include:

—Fibroids, or leiomyomata. These tumors, usually benign, occur most often in premenopausal women and recede after menopause when the ovaries are no longer producing estrogen, which in earlier years stimulated growth of the fibroid. Fibroids by themselves usually are *not* an indication for surgery. Surgery becomes necessary if they grow so large that they cause bladder or rectal problems, press on the ureters causing backup of urine into kidneys, or cause extreme pain or bleeding. In a young woman who may want to have children, a leiomyoma may be removed by myomectomy, a procedure in which a fibroid is shelled out of the uterine wall, leaving the uterus intact. Most physicians will recommend hysterectomy for symptomatic fibroids in women who have completed their families, although myomectomy can be considered at any age.

—Chronic infections. These usually cause chronic pain and often have recurrent flare-ups. Because women with chronic pelvic infections are often sterile due to blocked Fallopian tubes, some gynecology texts state that TAHBSO is the treatment of choice for recurrent symptomatic pelvic infection. For the individual woman who has been through a long period of chronic pain and recurrent illnesses from pelvic infections, hysterectomy may be a welcome solution.

—Chronic pelvic pain not caused by infections may necessitate hysterectomy after other methods of treatment have failed. Some women with crippling dysmenorrhea find hysterectomy the best solution to the severe menstrual pain. Endometriosis (uterine lining tissue outside the uterus) or adenomyosis (the same tissue within the muscular walls of the uterus) can cause cyclic pain that may not respond to mild pain medication. As we noted, fibroids or chronic infection can also cause pain. And pelvic pain, like any other type of pain, can, of course, be "functional" or emotional. But this diagnosis has been greatly overused in treatment of female complaints. Extreme stress being expressed as pelvic pain will not be helped by surgery, unless the stress is caused by recurrent pregnancy. Hysterectomy will cure *that* condition, but so will tubal ligation, which is simpler and easier.

—Uterine prolapse and "pelvic relaxation." Prolapse is a condition in which the uterus has weak tissue support and tends to slide down the vagina. In severe forms the uterus may literally fall out of the vagina. Pelvic relaxation refers to loosening of vaginal and uterine ligaments to the point where general vaginal laxity occurs. These conditions, which often occur together, may result from childbearing, obesity, poor tissue condition, advancing age or a combination of these. Historically, prolapse was treated with a variety of rather quaint pessaries (vaginal suppositories); and in the days of large families and poor obstetrical repair of tissues stretched and torn in childbirth, these conditions were very common. Now they are less common, but may still be a valid reason for surgery. Any woman who does not have symptoms or cannot actually feel her tissues "falling out" would do well to get a second opinion if told she needs surgery for "relaxation." On occasion, these conditions may cause painful intercourse or a sensation of a too loose vagina during intercourse; in these cases surgery may help.

—Cancer. In certain cases of Stage O (carcinoma in situ, i.e., localized) or Stage I cancer of the cervix, hysterectomy may be the procedure of choice. Endometrial cancer (of the lining of the uterus) is usually treated by hysterectomy and is sometimes preceded or followed by radiation to improve the results. Abdominal hysterectomy with the removal of tubes and ovaries, followed by radiation with or without chemotherapy, is the usual treatment for ovarian cancer. (See Chapter 14, "Cancer," for a discussion of these therapies.)

—Incontinence. (See later section in this chapter.)

—Sterilization. Hysterectomy is 100 percent effective in preventing pregnancy, but in the absence of other pelvic disease, simpler procedures (see tubal ligation in Chapter 7) are preferred.

Oophorectomy

Here we will examine the generally accepted practices regarding removal of the ovaries and then discuss some of the reasons this procedure is performed. Although there is much variation depending on the individual doctor and patient, the following guidelines may be used:

1. Ovaries are removed with hysterectomy in older women; physician opinion varies as to the age at which the ovaries should be removed.

2. Ovaries of young women are usually left in when hysterectomy is performed.

3. "Diseased" ovaries are usually removed at any age. They are also removed regardless of the woman's age in cases of hysterectomy for pelvic inflammatory disease, or in surgery for ovarian cysts or ectopic pregnancy when the ovary itself is not felt to be salvageable.

In older women ovaries are usually removed because of the risk of developing ovarian cancer (which can usually be detected only late in its course), and also because the ovaries are not believed necessary or functional in older women. The flaw in this theory is that the ovaries probably function to some degree until age sixty or more.

The concern about ovarian cancer is very real; one woman out of a hundred—amounting to some 10,000 women a year—will develop ovarian cancer; a large proportion of these will die from the disease.

Ovaries are usually left in a young woman because the ovaries are hormonally active during childbearing years, and it is generally believed that the body's own hormones are superior to prolonged use of hormone-replacement pills. Risks of long-term hormone replacement are unknown, but the dangers of severe menopausal symptoms, osteoporosis or premature aging in young women who are castrated and not given replacement hormones is felt to be great. However, in ovarian malignancy, severe pelvic inflammatory disease or diseases involving the ovaries, it is sometimes necessary to remove one or both ovaries at a young age. If this is done, replacement hormones should be taken at least until the time of normal menopause.

Appendectomy

Many gynecologists perform routine appendectomies during pelvic surgery on the theory that it may prevent the need for a later operation; many do not. If you care one way or the other, ask your surgeon before the operation what he normally does. Express your own feelings about whether an apparently healthy appendix should be removed. Obviously, if a diseased appendix is found (for example, during surgery for a suspected ectopic pregnancy), emergency removal is necessary.

Tubal Ligation. See Chapter 7.

Caesarean Section. See Chapter 6.

Dilation and Curettage (D&C)

In this procedure the mouth of the womb is held open so that a spoon-shaped instrument, the curette, can be inserted. The lining of the uterine wall is scraped in a systematic manner to ensure that no areas are missed.

The D&C is used both for diagnosis and for treatment. Causes of menstrual irregularities and abnormal postmenopausal bleeding may be sought by use of the D&C. It may also be used in treatment for heavy bleeding, incomplete abortion or to remove retained fragments of afterbirth following delivery. An early abortion may be performed by doing a D&C.

The "suction curettage" technique is similar to a D&C but uses a suction machine rather than a scraping tool. Suction is believed somewhat safer for early-pregnancy termination and miscarriage, but the D&C may be preferred for the more delicate tissues in a diagnostic procedure or immediately after childbirth. Either a local or a general anesthetic may be used. Many institutions now provide outpatient D&Cs.

Some conditions that once called for a D&C, such as unexplained bleeding or amenorrhea (absence of menstruation) in young women, may now be handled without hospitalization, with endometrial biopsy procedures and hormone treatment. At the present time, a D&C is necessary following most miscarriages. It is essential for postmenopausal women with unexplained bleeding because of the high risk in this age group of cancer that might not be detected by biopsy.

Surgery for Incontinence

Since the time of Dr. J. Marion Sims's experiments on slaves and poor New York immigrants, a great deal of surgical attention has been given to this very distressing condition, which can be personally and socially devastating. Urinary leakage can be caused by the stretching and tearing associated with childbirth, medical conditions like bladder infections or nervous instability of the bladder, or natural sagging of bladder support structures that can occur with advancing age and decreasing estrogens. Often a combination of factors is involved.

Before surgery is undertaken for correcting urinary incontinence, it is standard practice for the physician to test for possible diabetes, urinary-tract infection and nerve disorders, as well as to determine what is responsible structurally for the incontinence. This procedure usually includes a blood-sugar measurement, urine culture and a careful pelvic examination. It may also include cystometric studies of bladder capacity and function done with a urethral catheter and x-ray studies of bladder and kidneys. Sometimes the only treatment needed is antibiotics for a urinary-tract infection, estrogen cream for an atrophic (shrunken) vaginal and urethral opening, or medication for spasm of bladder muscles.

If surgery is necessary, the surgeon must choose from among a variety of procedures. If pressure from the uterus is complicating the problem, hysterectomy may be recommended. Most incontinence procedures involve one of these basic techniques:

1. The urethra is pulled up into a normal position by a sling, or stitching, procedure.

2. The vagina is "tightened" by removing wedges of stretched-out tissue and sewing the edges back together, putting the muscular and supporting tissues of the bladder and rectum back into their normal alignment.

The majority of women troubled by leaking urine can be cured by one of these procedures.

Rectal incontinence is even more distressing and debilitating. Although it is occasionally caused by nerve injury or nerve disease, it usually results from mechanical injury to the rectal muscles. Such injuries occur most commonly during childbirth. Barring the nerve disorders, effective treatment is a meticulous reconstruction of the normal muscle structures and attachments by a surgeon experienced in rectal surgery. As a last resort, colostomy (bringing the bowel out through an opening in the abdomen) may be necessary.

Infertility Surgery. See Chapter 8.

Laparoscopy

In this procedure a viewing instrument is inserted in an abdominal incision, usually just below the navel. Tubal ligations can be done in this manner, and laparoscopy is also often employed to diagnose suspected tubal pregnancy, infertility or chronic pelvic pain. Its advantages are that it is quick and relatively safe, and discloses a great deal of information about the condition of the pelvic organs without the scar formation and recovery time of a surgical exploration. It can be done on an outpatient basis, though most American hospitals are not prepared at present to handle minor outpatient surgery. Its disadvantages are that it requires fairly sophisticated equipment and a skilled laparoscopy/anesthesia team. There is risk of damage to pelvic organs during insertion of the laparoscope, complications that might require extensive surgery. In skilled hands, however, laparoscopy is quite safe and can often avert unnecessary surgery by allowing the surgeon to look at the pelvic organs through a tiny half-inch opening.

Salpingectomy

Removal of a Fallopian tube is generally done for a tubal pregnancy. This is a surgical emergency because the placental attachment will almost inevitably eat its way through the tube and lead to hemorrhage into the abdominal cavity. The surgeon rarely has any alternative to removing the tube, although occasionally it is possible to "milk" the pregnancy out of the tube. If you must undergo a salpingectomy, it is important for you to find out if the ovary was removed along with the tube, and also if the opposite tube was normal or appeared damaged. The condition of the opposite tube can determine your chances for a normal pregnancy, the possibilities of a fertility problem or the risk of tubal pregnancy on that side.

Breast Surgery

There are three major types of breast surgery: cancer surgery and reconstruction; augmentation surgery to enlarge breasts; and reduction surgery to correct oversized breasts.

Cancer surgery is discussed further in Chapter 14. It is important for the woman facing possible breast-cancer surgery to be aware of the medical controversy about treatment methods, involving radical mastectomy, simple mastectomy, or lumpectomy, all with or without adjuvant radiation therapy and chemotherapy (treatment with cancer drugs). There is still disagreement among cancer specialists about whether breast reconstruction should be done at all. Traditionally, it was believed that rebuilding the breast contour might mask a recurrence of cancer. This view has more or less been set aside, and recognition has grown of the tremendous psychological benefit of mammoplasty following, or performed along with, mastectomy.

If you have strong feelings on the subject, you would be wise to ask for a biopsy (under local anesthetic) of any breast lump before surgery is undertaken. If a malignancy is found, you may wish to gather several opinions before further surgery is scheduled.

Breast augmentation (or enlargement) can be done by several different techniques. Most often an inert implant (a soft plastic cushion) is slipped into the breast, leaving the nipple and some glandular tissue intact on top. Some women have even breast-fed infants after this procedure. For the woman with realistic expectations—larger breasts to look better beneath clothes—this procedure can be very satisfying.

In breast reduction, some of the fatty glandular tissue is removed. In most cases the surgeon tries to leave the nipple area intact. This operation can bring great relief for the woman with heavy, pendulous breasts that may cause back strain and shoulder pain. Clothes fit better, and good posture and a trim look are easier to attain. Again, esthetic perfection or repair of personal relationships is not guaranteed.

Check your insurance policy before having breast surgery. Many companies consider it "cosmetic" and will not pay the claim. You may decide to go ahead and pay for it on your own. Ask about surgeons' fees and expected hospitalization costs, but recognize that if complications arise, those costs may increase greatly. If you consider your surgery medically justified (for cancer reconstruction or a back condition), you may be able to claim insurance payment.

Of Special Concern When You Are Having Surgery

• *Legal issues.* There are two main legal issues you should understand. One is that the surgery must be authorized by the patient, and the other is that the surgery should be performed up to the standards of the medical profession for that procedure. A failure to perform up to professional standards constitutes negligence or malpractice. Let's look at the first requirement, which is sometimes called "informed consent." Before the patient can legally authorize the surgery, the patient must know and understand (1) what is to be done,

(2) the risks involved and (3) possible alternative treatments. Accordingly, before your surgery the physician will discuss all of these elements with you. You should feel free to ask any questions you have regarding any of these elements or any part of the surgery. When you are fully informed, you can give a proper authorization for the surgery. Although your verbal consent may be sufficient in some jurisdictions, in most places you will be asked to sign a form acknowledging that you have been given full information concerning your surgery and that you consent to the surgery.

The "informed consent" properly authorizes the physician to perform the surgery. Now the second element comes into play: The physician must perform the surgery so authorized with the degree of care and skill that the medical profession has established as the standard for physicians performing that procedure. People sometimes expect perfect results from surgery, and when the results are something less than the patient's expectations, the patient may feel that the doctor is liable for malpractice. However, even though the results of the surgery may not be "good," the physician has no legal liability as long as he performed the operation with that degree of care and skill established by the medical profession for that type of surgery. The physician cannot guarantee a perfect result and will be liable only if he was negligent in performing the surgery.

• *Routine tests.* On entering the hospital for surgery, you will probably be given blood tests, a chest x-ray and possibly an electrocardiogram. Routine preoperative tests have been criticized for being superfluous and an unnecessary expense. Hospitals are caught between trying to control costs and meeting the requirements of hospital accrediting agencies that call for certain pre-op tests. The individual patient has little control over the fact that the accrediting agency requires certain tests on all patients who are scheduled for surgery. These tests may safeguard the patient's health by making any abnormalities (which might otherwise go unrecognized) known to the anesthesiologist, the surgeon and the entire medical team.

• *Anesthesia.* For some procedures you may have a choice of a general, regional (such as spinal) or a local anesthetic. As a rule, regional and local anesthesia are considered safer than general anesthesia, which saturates heart and lung tissues with anesthetic agents. For some procedures, such as laparoscopy, regional anesthesia may not produce enough relaxation. For women with heart or serious lung disease, general anesthesia should be avoided if possible. If you have a preference in anesthesia, discuss it with your doctor before surgery. Your preference may be followed, though at times there are medical reasons for using one or another type of anesthesia.

• *Interns and residents.* Anyone who has had surgery in a teaching hospital has probably looked with some suspicion at the various young students and residents, thinking, just *who* is responsible for the surgery, anyway? In hospitals with no interns or residents, surgical assistants are employed to help with operations; in teaching hospitals, residents (doctors who are specialists-in-training) operate with the surgeons and assist while learning procedures. Indeed, on occasion a resident may do part or most of the operation, with your own surgeon being part of the team. If you trust your surgeon, it seems reasonable also to trust his assessment of an assistant's abilities. Resident participation in surgery is a fact of life at most teaching hospitals and has the advantage of round-the-clock coverage by a house medical staff. If you object strongly to interns and residents participating in your care, you should ask your surgeon to admit you to a hospital that does not have residents.

• *After your surgery.* Having made it through the blur of your postoperative hospitalization—the "cough, turn, deep-breathe, have-you-moved-your-bowels-yet" and the liquid-to-bland-to-solid diet routine—you may find some lingering problems. Most people, after coming home from the hospital, experience some strange and worrisome difficulties but feel awkward about calling the doctor. Let's talk about some of them:

—Pain. Surgical trauma, the injury and insult to tissues during surgery, does cause pain. After a D&C or a miscarriage many women have cramps for a few days. After major surgery, soreness around the incision and in the related muscles is normal for several weeks. But sudden, excruciating pain or pain accompanied by fever or heavy bleeding should receive medical attention.

—Bleeding. A certain amount of bleeding is natural after pelvic surgery. The small amount of blood that escapes from affected tissues may exit from the vagina. As a rule of thumb, if bleeding is not heavier than a period and seems to be diminishing in flow, it is probably normal. But a sudden heavy flow of bright-red blood or bleeding accompanied by dizziness, fainting or chills calls for prompt medical investigation.

—Fever. Fever following a surgical procedure can signal wound infection. It should be evaluated medically as soon as possible.

—Sexual intercourse. After most pelvic surgery, women are generally warned not to have intercourse until after a postoperative checkup. After a D&C, the purpose of temporary abstinence is to avoid spreading infection up the still abnormally dilated cervix and into the uterus. After hysterectomy, there may be the danger of tearing open stitches, which could lead to infection or hemorrhage. Ask your doctor about the advisable interval before resuming intercourse.

Dyspareunia, or painful intercourse, is commonly noted by women after pelvic surgery. Some physicians believe this complaint is largely psychological, but it is more realistic to ascribe dyspareunia to physical reasons. There is recent tissue trauma; there is scar tissue; and there may be some shortening of the vagina or change in the natural angle of the vagina. There may be disruption of normal secretions with a fall in estrogen levels, resulting in thinning and fragility of vaginal walls. Finally, there may be some changes in vaginal size and resiliency caused by temporary disuse during the period of surgery.

Most of these problems are correctable. The vagina is highly elastic, and with repeated intercourse or through stretching with vaginal dilators, the painful effects of scar tissue or vaginal shortening can be eliminated. Lubricants and estrogen therapy can counteract the missing secretions or natural estrogens. It may take work to bring back full and comfortable sexual function, but the postoperative woman owes it to herself and her partner to return to satisfying sexual activity. Postoperative dyspareunia should not be viewed as permanent. Be sure to let your doctor know if you are having any problems with intercourse so that you can get all the help available.

—Fatigue. This is *normal!* Anyone who undergoes major surgery is likely to feel tired and to need extra rest for several months, so do not fret if you don't feel "back to your old self" the minute you get home. The postoperative period is an ideal time to concentrate on good habits of rest, exercise and nutrition.

—Depression. The "post-hysterectomy blues" has often been labeled as the usual female neurosis. There is nothing neurotic about depression following female surgery. It is a perfectly normal mourning process. In hysterectomy or mastectomy, a woman has lost an organ which our society equates with feminine value. Loss of a female organ can have a profound effect on her body image and feelings of self-worth.

Not only must the post-op woman work through her own feelings, but those of her husband or partner, her children, and her friends and relatives. All of these persons may react with fear and worry over her illness. Added to these readjustment problems are the burdens of normal postoperative fatigue, possibly premature menopause, time lost from work, and often a financial strain from medical bills. Depression is easy to understand.

The woman who has had cancer surgery bears a very special burden. First, she must face the terror of her own impending mortality. This may be coupled with the loneliness of being unable to share her fears and bitterness with those close to her who assert jubilantly, "You should be grateful that you may be cured."

Most women depend on supportive friends while working out these understandable feelings of depression. Supportive male figures can be helpful, but often husbands or partners have their own set of fears and adjustments to handle. If you must adjust to major surgery, you may derive great benefit from an organization of fellow former patients.

The wonder is not that women suffer postsurgical depression but that virtually all of them successfully get through the temporary depression to reach a new level of self-esteem and a new realization of the strength of their own femininity.

11

GYNECOLOGIC SYMPTOMS: WHAT DO THEY MEAN, WHAT SHOULD YOU DO?

Gone are the days when the mere fact of womanhood implied sickness, when pregnancy and menstrual periods were universally considered illnesses. Gone also is the notion that any time illness strikes a female, it is necessarily a "female" illness. Under that distorted doctrine, when a woman came down with anything—from tuberculosis to intestinal disease—it was attributed to a disorder of her uterus. These assumptions made it difficult if not impossible to identify and treat either a body disorder not involving the genital tract or a primarily gynecologic problem.

In Chapter 4 we discussed general physical symptoms, along with some approaches to understanding and dealing with them effectively. Certain gynecologic symptoms have already been discussed in the preceding chapters on menstruation, pregnancy, contraception and infections; now let's talk briefly about some general abdominal-pain problems before we get to the most commonly encountered gynecologic symptoms, what they mean, and how you should handle them.

Abdominal Pain—Nongynecologic Causes

Probably the most important fact to remember is that there are a lot of structures in the abdomen besides the uterus, tubes and ovaries, and that the gastrointestinal (GI) system can cause a wide variety of types of abdominal pain. Ulcer disease often causes sharp pains in the upper abdomen varying with food intake. Liver disease or pancreatic disease may cause an ill-defined abdominal pain. Gallstones or inflammatory gall-bladder disease typically causes pain in the right upper part of the abdomen, sometimes accompanied by digestive disturbances.

Simple gas pains can cause a great deal of discomfort almost anywhere in the abdomen. Inflammatory bowel disease can cause varied types of abdominal discomfort, which may be localized in the right lower part of the abdomen, as in Crohn's disease, or in the left side, as in ulcerative colitis. Appendicitis is classically described as a sharp, lower right abdominal pain, but it may begin in the area of the navel. During pregnancy, appendicitis may cause pain in the right upper part of the abdomen because the appendix is pushed upward by the enlarging uterus. Previous abdominal surgery can cause scar tissue or adhesions in the abdomen. These may result in chronic pain or even in the surgical emergency of a bowel obstruction.

The urinary-tract organs can also cause symptoms that may be misdiagnosed as "female problems." Cystitis, or a bladder infection, may cause low pelvic discomfort. Back pain or abdominal pain may result from either cystitis or a more serious kidney infection (pyelonephritis). Kidney stones may cause excruciating pain in the back or pelvis. And while we're on the subject of lower-back pain we should note that disk problems or typical lower-back strain can occur in women as easily as in men. Gone are the days of attributing back pain in women to a "tipped uterus" without considering the possibility of a back problem.

The point here is not to list every disorder imaginable, but to illustrate the variety of medical dysfunctions that may cause abdominal pain besides gynecologic problems. When you are seeking a medical opinion about abdominal pain, whether from a gynecologist, internist or emergency-room physician, be ready to supply information about any recent discomfort after eating or any recent exposure to infections (such as travel in countries where hepatitis or parasites are endemic). The examining physician will probably question you about digestive and urinary function and do a careful general exam of your entire abdomen. He may also ask about recent periods, contraceptive practice and recent sexual activity.

Pelvic Pain—Gynecologic Causes

Many conditions can cause pelvic pain. Types of pain can be loosely organized into groupings based on the circumstances surrounding the pain, such as whether it is related to pregnancy or whether it is accompanied by fever or chills. You should always remember that pelvic pain can be a great "mimicker" and that symptoms can vary widely with different conditions.

MENSTRUAL PAIN

Plain old-fashioned cramps have been given the fancier name "dysmenorrhea" in medical circles. For hundreds of years or more, women were alternately told that cramps were "all in your mind" *or* that cramps were so debilitating that women should not be allowed to perform work requiring any kind of responsibility. Whether cramps were considered emotionally based or physically disabling depended on whether the woman was expected to work for a living or was considered uppity and trying to encroach on male territory. Only in the late 1970s was it discovered that, when the actual pressure of cramps was measured, in many cases women with severe dysmenorrhea experienced cramps stronger than labor pains. The chemical culprits in dysmenorrhea are prostaglandins, substances made in the uterus that cause constriction of blood vessels and painful cramps. Fortunately there are several effective medications on the market that specifically inhibit the formation or action of prostaglandins. Plain aspirin is a weak prostaglandin inhibitor; many over-the-counter medicines containing aspirin are effective in treating mild cramps.

Many women experience a more general "premenstrual syndrome" just before and during menses. This may include a bloated sensation and weight gain due to fluid retention, headache, and emotional ups and downs. Occasionally a diuretic is necessary to get rid of excess fluid, but generally just being aware that this syndrome is a part of the normal cycle will help you be philosophical about it. Try to get some extra rest, and remember that this monthly "down" is *not* a time of total incapacity or a time when women cannot handle important tasks. Most women learn to live with their periods, and given proper treatment for medically disabling headaches, dysmenorrhea and fluid retention, there are few who cannot maintain their topnotch working level every day of the month.

Endometriosis can cause severe pain preceding menstruation. The bleeding that occurs with menstruation from this displaced tissue can cause severe dysmenorrhea, as well as dyspareunia (painful intercourse) and infertility.

There are several approaches to treatment of endometriosis. For some women, hormone manipulation with estrogens and progestins, sometimes called "pseudopregnancy," are effective. For a woman who does not want to get pregnant, low-dose oral contraceptive pills may relieve the pain of endometriosis by gradually reducing the thickness and amount of bleeding from the endometrial tissue in the pelvis. Many women who have endometriosis do not have severe pain and can use mild analgesics as needed.

Women with severe pain who also want sterilization may have a hysterectomy, along with removal of the abnormal endometrial-like tissue. Women who want to remain fertile may be able to have a meticulous excision of the abnormal tissue that leaves reproductive structures intact.

The less common condition called adenomyosis is the presence of endometrial tissue within the muscular layer of the uterus, the myometrium. Cyclic menstrual bleeding into the myometrium can be extremely painful. Sometimes this pain can be controlled by one of the above measures. Hysterectomy may be needed if the condition does not respond to hormonal or analgesic therapy and is truly disabling.

PAIN WITH INTERCOURSE (DYSPAREUNIA)

This condition can have a drastic effect on a woman's sexual relationships and hence on her self-image and her self-esteem. Fortunately, during the past twenty years we have come a long way in understanding the causes of dyspareunia and in developing effective treatments. Dyspareunia is a common, generally treatable symptom, and a woman experiencing discomfort with intercourse should not hesitate to seek medical advice.

Two basic types of dyspareunia are pain on entry into the vagina, usually due to local vaginal problems, and pain on deep penetration, which is due to problems within the inner pelvic organs. Vaginal pain may be due to vaginitis of almost any type. (See Chapter 9 on infections.) Vaginitis due to local infections can generally be treated with local or systemic antibiotics. Atrophic vaginitis (irritation from shrunken vaginal tissues), which usually occurs in older women, is easily cured by estrogen in either cream or pill form. Estrogens are critical in giving the vaginal tissues thickness and resiliency; loss of estrogenic support can cause thinning, tenderness and fragility of the vaginal tissues, making intercourse painful. Lacerations of the vagina during childbirth, if not properly repaired, can result in dyspareunia. (See Chapter 10 for measures to improve postoperative vaginal function.)

Vaginismus (a spasm of the vaginal muscles that results in pain on attempting intercourse) has received a great deal of attention from sex therapists. Most women will experience vaginismus at some point in their lives, perhaps when they are first having intercourse, or when they are upset and not in the mood for intercourse, or after a traumatic experience such as rape. For a fair number of women, involuntary vaginismus can cause chronic sexual problems. For a long time, vaginismus was considered to be a purely psychological problem, and women were sent to psychotherapists. Now, however, it is recognized that for many women painful experiences during intercourse set off a vicious circle resulting in the *expectation* of pain to the point where involuntary vaginal muscle spasms make intercourse even more painful. For these women, optimal treatment consists of self-exploration and vaginal manipulation, often with dilators, so that they can learn to relax and unlearn the responses that resulted in vaginismus.

Pain occurring with deep thrusting movements by the man during intercourse usually points to a problem with the uterus or deep tissues of the pelvis. Endometriosis, as mentioned previously, can cause dyspareunia. Uterine fibroids or adenomyosis may be tender and cause pain when the uterus is moved about during intercourse. Pelvic infections, scar tissue from adhesions, or ovarian cysts may cause uncomfortable intercourse. Unfortunately, treatment for these conditions is not always successful. Physicians may recommend hysterectomy for fibroids, inflammatory disease or other conditions that cause severe dyspareunia. In many cases, such surgery will alleviate the pain.

PREGNANCY-RELATED PELVIC PAIN

Normal pregnancy can be uncomfortable. Early in pregnancy many women experience a fullness and aching sensation in the lower abdomen, often accompanied by frequent urination. At three to four months gestation many women experience a tugging sensation at the sides called "round ligament pain." It is attributed to the stretching of these ligaments, two rounded cords between the supportive layers of the broad ligaments in the abdomen. Throughout pregnancy most women experience abdominal discomfort due to gas and constipation. Many women develop quite debilitating back pain due to the weight of the baby and the postural lordosis (swayback) that occurs late in pregnancy; at the same time, pressure from the baby's head may cause pain on the pubic bone. And finally, intermittent contractions (called Braxton-Hicks contractions) often occur during the last few weeks of pregnancy; many women do not find these small contractions painful, but for some women (particularly teenagers) these can be frightening and quite uncomfortable.

Miscarriage causes rather distinctive cramping pelvic pain. Since a large percentage of early miscarriages are due to genetic abnormalities in the fetus, physicians rarely try to stop them, merely advising bed rest when severe cramps herald a spontaneous abortion. Later in pregnancy, however (about twenty weeks, or sometimes "viability" at about twenty-eight weeks), most physicians try to stop the process of miscarriage, which is called "premature labor." Therefore, if you experience cramps early in pregnancy, there is really no point in rushing to the hospital, since little will be done unless heavy bleeding accompanies the cramps. If you experience regular, frequent contractions after your fourth month of pregnancy, you should seek medical attention quickly because it is better to stop premature labor before dilation of the cervix has occurred.

Ectopic pregnancy (pregnancy outside the uterus) is a medical emergency. In approximately one out of 100 pregnancies, the fertilized egg implants itself outside of the uterine cavity. Usually this occurs when the Fallopian tubes have been damaged by infection or scar tissue. Most often the egg will become implanted in the Fallopian tube, but the egg can alight on any structure in the abdomen. Initially the fertilized egg starts to grow, sending tendrils of placental tissue invading the structure on which it has landed. Usually within the first six to eight weeks of pregnancy, these invading tendrils will rupture into blood vessels, causing bleeding that can quickly turn into intra-abdominal hemorrhage.

The first signs (there are many) of ectopic pregnancy include abnormal bleeding and one-sided abdominal pain. Since women who develop ectopic pregnancy often have a history of pelvic inflammatory disease (PID), their complaints of pain may be attributed to recurrent PID, and the possibility of ectopic pregnancy could be overlooked. Women with IUDs in place are also more likely to develop ectopic pregnancies. If the condition is diagnosed at the first complaint of pelvic pain, an ectopic pregnancy can be removed before it ruptures and bleeds.

Often an ectopic pregnancy is found only after hemorrhage has occurred and the woman arrives at the hospital in shock. Since very few conditions other than ectopic pregnancy cause an otherwise healthy young woman to suddenly collapse in shock from blood loss, the diagnosis can quickly be made and emergency surgery performed. Virtually the only treatment for ectopic pregnancy is removal of the pregnancy. If a woman is not in shock, and ectopic pregnancy is suspected, many doctors will perform a laparoscopy (see Chapter 10) for diagnosis, and if an ectopic gestation is found, proceed immediately to opening the abdomen and removing the pregnancy. When the pregnancy is in a Fallopian tube, that tube must almost always be removed, although occasionally a surgeon can "milk" out the gestational sac and leave the tube intact. More often, however, the tube is irreparably damaged by the ectopic pregnancy and would be useless, anyway. If the tube on the opposite side is all right, prospects for normal future pregnancies are excellent. Unfortunately, the opposite tube is sometimes diseased as a result of the infection or the damage that caused the first tube to harbor an ectopic gestation.

Ectopic pregnancy has been called "the great mimicker" because its symptoms can simulate almost any other abdominal condition— appendicitis, PID and ovarian cysts among others. Any persistent abdominal pain, particularly if one-sided, in a potentially pregnant woman merits medical attention. The patient should be very open with the examining doctor about any unprotected intercourse, any missed periods and any history of pelvic infections. There are few diagnoses more difficult to make than that of early ectopic pregnancy, and few diagnoses that are easier to miss.

OVARIAN CYSTS

These growths are common. In young women the majority of ovarian growths are benign cysts. However, in older women, past the age of ovulation, a good proportion of ovarian masses will be cancerous. (See Chapter 14 for discussion of ovarian cancers.)

There are several types of benign ovarian cysts. The most common is the follicular cyst, which merely represents an enlarged egg-producing follicle that for some unknown reason fills with fluid. Corpus-luteum cysts may result when a follicle releases an egg and then enlarges; normally corpus-luteum cysts measure one inch, but on occasion they may become "persistent" and enlarge to two inches and produce symptoms.

The majority of corpus-luteum and follicular cysts will disappear spontaneously, so that it is common practice for physicians to wait and re-examine a young woman two or more weeks after a cyst is found to see if it has dissolved by itself. If the cyst is persistent over several weeks, or if a cyst is causing symptoms, or if the physician has any reason to suspect a possible tubal pregnancy, surgical exploration is also advisable. In an older woman, any ovarian enlargement makes surgical exploration necessary because of the high risk of malignancy.

In addition to corpus-luteum and follicular cysts, women can develop a number of other types of ovarian cysts. One of the more interesting types is called a "dermoid." Dermoid cysts are benign growths containing mixed-up bits of mature human tissue. They may contain skin, hair, cartilage—and even well-formed teeth! They require surgery, since dermoids, like any type of cyst, may twist and cause severe pain. In general, dermoids can be removed, leaving behind a normal ovary and allowing for normal future fertility. Left untreated, most cysts will rupture and bleed, or twist and cause severe pain. Cysts must be removed and checked to make sure they are not malignant and that the mass felt is not an ectopic pregnancy, abscess or other pelvic tumor.

TOXIC SHOCK SYNDROME

Late in the summer of 1980 what looked like a new disease, toxic shock syndrome (TSS), appeared at rapidly increasing rates in scattered locations throughout America. The infection, which almost always struck women during a menstrual period, would bring on a sudden high fever with a severe drop in blood pressure. Other symptoms were vomiting, diarrhea and a rash that later peeled off in scales. The disease was evidently associated with the use of tampons. Researchers soon isolated the common infectious organism *Staphylococcus aureus* and declared it to be the cause—which deepened the mystery because aureus-infection sites are traditionally skin, bone or respiratory areas, not the vagina.

By late autumn, hundreds of cases were reported to the government's Center for Disease Control, with an alarming 10 percent death rate. One tampon brand was withdrawn from the market by its manufacturers when researchers found that it was used by more than seven out of ten women who came down with TSS. The American College of Obstetricians and Gynecologists advised women to stop using "super absorbent" types of tampons until further studies could be done. "In general, women need not stop using tampons," said the ACOG statement. But several of the newest types of tampons designed for super absorbency contain special synthetic fibers that may very well create conditions favorable to the growth of the infectious organism or enable it to produce increased amounts of toxins, the poisonous by-product that may cause symptoms. Those conditions have yet to be discovered. Some types of fiber used in tampons may act to dam the menstrual flow too much, creating an effective culture environment for the organism. Many physicians and ACOG recommend that tampons be changed frequently to prevent this condition—at least every four to six hours. To further reduce risk, alternate tampons with sanitary napkins or mini-pads.

It is also possible that scratching of the vaginal surface either by the tampons themselves or by the plastic applicators used for inserting them is a source of the disorder. If this is indeed one reason, then changing tampons too frequently may actually increase the risk.

As this is written, scientists are investigating an antitoxin that may be used for vaccination against the disease. Tampon packages contain information that gives details about symptoms, and instructions on medical help in case a problem occurs.

Meanwhile, if you become ill with a fever, vomiting, diarrhea or a sunburnlike rash during a menstrual period—especially if you use tampons—see a doctor at once. There are effective antibiotics for TSS.

PELVIC INFECTIONS

Pelvic infections are a common cause of pain; pelvic inflammatory disease (PID) may indeed be *the* most common cause of pelvic pain seen in most hospital emergency rooms. As a result, many other conditions may be misdiagnosed as PID. Details of PID are covered in Chapter 9; here we shall merely discuss the type of pain it causes.

The "classical" attack of PID occurs right after a menstrual period (when, evidently, infectious organisms can spread up the uterus into the Fallopian tubes) and consists of bilateral low pelvic pain, fever and often a foul vaginal discharge. Walking or any type of motion is exquisitely painful, resulting in a hunched-over, shuffling type of a gait jokingly dubbed in many emergency rooms the "PID shuffle." After recurrent attacks, abscess formation can occur in the areas of tubes and ovaries, resulting in a more severe, one-sided pain, frequently accompanied by peritonitis and debilitating illness. More often, a continual syndrome of low pelvic pain called "chronic PID" may develop, aggravated by intercourse and often associated with infertility. These problems frequently occur after repeated gonorrhea infections, but in many cases appendicitis, postpartum infections, or viral or chlamydial infections, rather than "VD" types of infections, can cause pelvic inflammatory disease. Treatment for uncomplicated cases may consist of antibiotic therapy. Unfortunately, severe, recurrent PID may require surgery, often hysterectomy. (See Chapter 10.) PID, with or without surgery, will often render a woman sterile by causing damage to the Fallopian tubes.

Dysmenorrhea, endometriosis, infections, cysts and pregnancy-related problems account for most true gynecologic pain. Any pain you cannot attribute to physiologic causes, such as menstruation, ovulation or normal pregnancy-related pain, deserves investigation. But be prepared for a long and arduous process—unless a very obvious abnormality is found. Detecting or diagnosing the cause of pelvic pain can be a difficult task, and treating it successfully more difficult still.

Abnormal Vaginal Bleeding

Menstrual-flow disorders (which we have discussed in detail in Chapter 5), include too much or too little bleeding. If you have either condition, your physician should investigate it. Heavy bleeding is likely to indicate a disorder that needs treatment, and if neglected, it can keep you anemic and susceptible to many problems such as infections. Scanty or missing periods may show that your endocrine system isn't functioning properly. Both conditions can be caused by, or result in, various problems of general health or they can be related to problems originating elsewhere in your body.

Nonmenstrual bleeding from the vagina must be investigated every time it occurs. Bleeding can be one sign of cancer, but more often it is not, so there's no need to panic at the sight of blood. Among the most common causes of nonmenstrual bleeding are dryness of the vagina; slight injuries sustained during intercourse; uterine polyp (a benign growth that's readily removed by surgery and tends not to come back); infection—and, of course, pregnancy.

Unexpected vaginal bleeding in older women must always be followed up medically. The risk of gynecologic cancer is greater after menopause. Expected or induced bleeding from cyclic estrogen replacement therapy is, of course, quite all right.

Vaginal Discharge

If the discharge is unusually profuse, and smells bad, or if you itch, get medical help. The cause may be a vaginal infection (see Chapter 9), a noninfectious irritation or a growth setting up an inflammation. But remember that some vaginal secretion is perfectly normal. Also, it may become a bit generous at times during the menstrual cycle, with sexual excitement or with oral contraceptives.

Abdominal Bloating, Stuffiness, Heavy Feeling

A heavy, puffy feeling is a common experience during the ovulation cycle. Many women have transient weight gains of several pounds at mid-cycle, all of it accounted for by retained fluid. (See Chapter 5 for more about this.)

A heavy feeling in the pelvis unexplained by cyclic events is sometimes the major symptom for any of several displacement disorders of the genital tract. Conditions whose names end in *-cele*, which means hernia, are more common in older women than in younger women, but may also follow childbirth or any injury that weakens internal support structures. Rectocele is a bulging of the rectum up through the vaginal wall. In cystocele, the bladder pushes in the vaginal wall. Urethrocele, or displacement of the urethral tubes, may cause involuntary dribbling or leakage of urine, a condition called stress incontinence.

The physician may give a series of training sessions on control of the stream of urine, helping the patient to regain tone of the sphincter, the closure muscle. Another corrective measure is surgery. Prolapse of the uterus, which drops toward the introitus, or vaginal opening, is also correctable by surgery. (See Chapter 10.)

Breast Symptoms

Sore and swollen breasts are very familiar to most women as just another mid-cycle or premenstrual signal. Breasts may become painful during pregnancy, of course, while they're preparing for lactation. In such instances a firm, supportive brassiere can be comforting.

When breasts become sore or swollen unexpectedly, and the symptom is not due to menstruation or pregnancy, medical attention is a must. Mastitis, or breast infection, can cause sore, swollen breasts. Drainage from the breast may signal an abscess. Generally, mastitis and breast abscesses occur in conjunction with pregnancy; they can almost always be treated with antibiotics. Breast lumps are benign about 80 percent of the time. Many women have a chronic condition called fibrocystic breast disease, which is noncancerous, although incidence of breast cancer is somewhat higher in women with benign breast disease. Recently some medical researchers claimed that complete abstinence from coffee, tea, chocolate and cola drinks will provide relief to some women with cystic breasts; a chemical family called xanthines, of which caffeine is a member, was thought to stimulate the breast condition. One study indicated that eliminating xanthines from the diet will prevent breast soreness. Some researchers feel that oral contraceptives reduce the incidence of fibrocystic disease.

The data are not conclusive; at present they point to the pill as a useful contraceptive agent for women with fibrocystic disease. Women with extremely fibrocystic breasts must often undergo instrument biopsy or needle biopsy (withdrawal of the fluid by needle) to ensure that all breast nodules are benign.

The Abnormal Pap Smear

Women may be confused and unnecessarily frightened about having an "abnormal Pap smear." The confusion is understandable, because an abnormal Pap smear may mean one of several things. Treatment will depend upon the age and reproductive wishes of the individual woman, as well as on the degree of the Pap-smear abnormality.

A Pap smear consists of cell scrapings from the vaginal walls and the cervix. (See illustration). Abnormalities that can be revealed by a Pap smear include cervicitis (inflammation of the cervix), dysplasia (abnormal surface tissue), carcinoma in situ (localized cancer) and invasive cervical cancer. Pap smears are "graded" on a scale of one to four or five, with Class I representing normal cells, Class II inflammatory changes, and Classes III to IV or V representing increasing degrees of abnormality and obviously malignant cells.

For chronic inflammation, most physicians will treat any infections when they occur, and repeat the Pap smear at regular and frequent intervals. If the smear does not indicate improvement, a physician may recommend cryosurgery (freezing), cauterization (burning), laser therapy, or even conization (removal of a cone-shaped piece of the cervix) to remove the abnormal inflammatory

PAP SMEAR

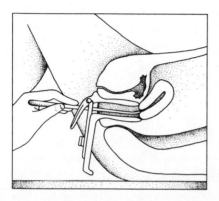 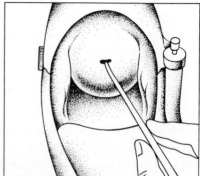

How the Pap test is done: *Cross section from the side shows the vaginal speculum in place. Sample of surface cells is taken by gently scraping the vaginal wall. Sample is also taken from the cervical opening. Sampling may cause a very small amount of bleeding but is not painful.*
Scraped-off cells are spread on a glass slide and treated with fixative (which could be plain hairspray), then stained to make them clearly visible under the microscope.
Head-on view of the cervix shows what physician or nurse practitioner sees when taking a Pap smear. Instrument is collecting sample from the endocervix (just inside the mouth of the cervix), where part of the Pap smear and cultures for a gonorrhea test are taken.

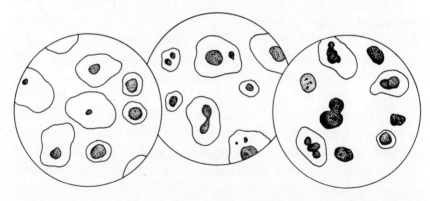

Seen under microscope. *Normal cervical cells* (left) *are large and pale, with a small nucleus. Cervical dysplasia* (center) *may yield cells with a larger or odd-shaped nucleus. Typical cancer cells* (right) *may have a bizarre nucleus, and they lose their pale, regular appearance. Interpretation is made only after examination of all cells of a smear.*

cells and promote formation of a new, healthy layer of cells on the cervix. Since chronic cervicitis may precede the development of cancer, a persistent Class II Pap smear deserves close attention.

Dysplasia, or the occurrence of abnormal cells suggestive of "precancerous" cells, is one of the most controversial areas of medicine. Dysplasias are separated into "mild," "moderate" and "severe," with mild dysplasias being treated more like chronic cervicitis, and severe dysplasias more like early carcinoma in situ. The basic problem in treating dysplasias is that with no treatment at all, roughly one fourth of them will get better, one fourth of them will get worse (become carcinoma in situ or frank invasive cancer) and one half of them will not change at all. Because of their high risk of developing into cancer, most dysplasias merit some type of medical treatment, which may vary with the woman, her physician and the exact nature of the cervical lesion. Here are some of the types of treatment used:

1. *Careful observation.* A very mild dysplasia may be watched carefully, with frequent Pap smears; possibly colposcopy and biopsy.

2. *Colposcopy.* An office procedure using a telescope-like machine that simply magnifies the view of the cervix through a regular speculum. With the colposcope, a physician may get a good look at the affected parts of the cervix, and may perform a biopsy on the areas that are abnormal. However, colposcopy requires special training and equipment and may not be available in all areas.

3. *Cautery and cryosurgery.* Cautery, or "burning," and cryosurgery, or "freezing," the cervix may be used to destroy abnormal tissue and promote healing with new, normal tissue. They can generally be done in the doctor's office, avoiding the expense of hospitalization. Cautery and cryosurgery should only be done after the cervix has been thoroughly evaluated with Pap smears, biopsy, and possibly colposcopy. The danger of these techniques is that they may "bury" an early, treatable cancer.

4. *Biopsy.* Cervical biopsy may also be performed as an office procedure to evaluate the severity of an abnormal Pap smear. Although the smear is an excellent screening test to detect abnormal cells, an actual chunk of tissue is much more reliable in determining the extent of the abnormality.

5. *Cervical conization.* This is a procedure that involves removing a circular cone-shaped piece of the cervix. This serves a dual purpose: It removes the actual cells and allows the pathologists to evaluate the depth of the abnormal cells; therefore, it may cure the abnormality and at the same time preserve childbearing function. Conization may also be done prior to a hysterectomy to make certain that there is no invading cancer, which would require different treatment. When conization is performed in a young woman who desires a family, there is a small risk of later infertility due to changes in the cervix. (The risk of infertility also exists, however, with cryosurgery and cautery). But since the risk of infertility is small and the risk of cancer from severe dysplasia is significant, conization may be strongly recommended for severe dysplasia.

6. *Hysterectomy.* For women who have completed their families, hysterectomy is often advised when the Pap smear shows serious dysplasia. Women seeking tubal ligations may be advised to have a hysterectomy instead if their Pap smears show dysplastic changes. This is a controversial area. For women with very mild dysplasia, a hysterectomy is probably not necessary; women with severe dysplasia or carcinoma in situ may be well advised to have a hysterectomy to prevent further problems. But for the gray area in the middle, no consensus exists, and the decision for or against hysterectomy will depend upon the individual woman and her physician. If you are in doubt, a second medical opinion may help you in deciding whether to have surgery.

Carcinoma in situ (CIS) is a premalignant lesion and requires aggressive therapy to prevent the development of cancer. In carcinoma in situ, malignant-appearing cells occupy the entire surface layer of the cervix. Traditionally, CIS has been treated in one of two ways: conization for young women who want to have children, and hysterectomy for women with no interest in future childbearing. There have always been a few advocates of cryosurgery or cautery, and more recently, of laser therapy for CIS. The problem with cryosurgery and cautery is that while they may destroy the top layer of cells on the cervix, they do not allow for careful inspection of the underlying cells to be sure that no malignant cells have been left behind. With the laser beam, actual cervical conization may be performed, and the underlying cells removed for inspection.

At present, laser treatment is available only in a few specialized centers and does not offer any obvious advantages over the traditional conization techniques, although future experience may prove it to be a preferred method for CIS and dysplasias. Anyone who is treated for CIS must have careful follow-up.

Dysplasia and CIS are part of a continuum referred to as intraepithelial neoplasia or CIN. While it is not an overt malignancy, women with any form of CIN are at risk and should have frequent exams and Pap smears no matter what type of treatment they have had. With careful medical follow-up, women with CIN should rarely have to worry about developing a serious cancer, but they should realize that hysterectomy or surgical conization may become necessary and plan their families accordingly. (See Chapter 14 for a discussion of cervical cancer.)

A great deal of controversy has recently centered around the question of how often women should have a Pap smear. The Pap smear is one of the most effective cancer-screening devices ever created, protecting women by early detection from developing cervical cancer (but *not* other types of gynecologic malignancy). Since the advent of the Pap smear, the death rate from cervical cancer has steadily decreased, and advanced cervical cancer, which once was the most common killer among gynecologic cancers, is a rarity among women who have regular Pap smears.

Cervical cancers develop slowly as a rule, and there is usually a ten- to-fifteen-year period between the development of dysplasia, CIS and cervical cancer. Furthermore, cervical cancer rarely develops in women who have had perfectly normal Pap smears over the course of several years. As a result, the American Cancer Society at one point recommended yearly Pap smears but later changed the recommendation to Pap smears at three-year intervals for women with no history of abnormal Pap smears. But most gynecologists are strongly opposed to the less frequent Pap smears. For the woman who develops a malignancy in a three-year interval, cost saving would be little consolation if yearly smears might have detected her cancer in time for cure. Furthermore, yearly gynecologic exams may detect other problems at an early, treatable stage. Finally, we all know that we tend to put off visits to the doctor: one-year

intervals become a little longer, and three-year intervals may become five-year intervals. The very women who should get frequent
checkups are the ones most likely to space out their exams. As a
result of these considerations, most doctors will continue to recommend yearly Pap smears; and you can bet that most women doctors
will be getting their own Pap smears done every year.

PART III

MATURITY: WELL–BEING PAST CHILDBEARING

"They don't make mirrors the way they used to."

—*overheard*

From about our mid-thirties on, we are in the mature phase of life
—"grown up at last," as you sometimes hear it expressed. There's
no guarantee, of course, of maturity in terms of behavior or outlook;
that's an attainment which is strictly up to each of us as an individual.

In this section we will explore the climacteric, that stage of a
woman's life which follows the childhood years and the fertile years.
In its Greek source, the word "climacteric" refers to a rung of a
ladder, *klimakter,* with the clear implication, in personal terms, that
a person has attained a certain level.

From that level, let's look around us.

Menopause—the cessation of the menses—is predominant as the
central happening of this phase. Yet it's a phase that often amounts
to a large portion of a woman's lifetime. Does it make sense, you
may ask, to label so many precious years "postmenopausal"? Isn't
this a simplistic distortion of an individual's life? There are at least
three major factors that help explain why we tend to exaggerate
menopause as a life event.

One is that medical practice and research define menopause as a
health problem—and not surprisingly so, since doctors mainly see
those women who are having problems.

The next, and perhaps the underlying factor, is that folklore
identifies and evaluates women by their reproductive functions; and

certainly, during the nineteenth century and in much of this one, medicine perpetuated the stereotype. If bearing (and incidentally rearing) children is the only valuable thing a woman can do, small wonder that she is relegated to the social scrap heap when her childbearing days are over.

Perhaps the heaviest item we must remove from society's load of ill-conceived notions is this triple-headed monster:

> Menstruation is illness.
> Pregnancy is illness.
> Menopause is illness.

There are indeed disorders and medical considerations related to each gynecologic function, just as there are in breathing, digestion and the circulation of the blood. In the chapters that follow, we will first take up the physiology of the climacteric years, which includes the changes of aging, with menopause as only one part of the process. Then come diet, exercise and sexuality as they affect the mature woman, with special emphasis on self-care and self-knowledge. Finally, we will discuss cancers in women, particularly of the reproductive tract and breasts. This important chapter is placed in the section of the book that is devoted to the older woman not because cancer is limited to this age group, but because its incidence is higher in the mature years.

12

"THE CHANGE OF LIFE"

"Progressive changes that take place in a cell, an organ, or the total person with the passage of time"—that is how the *Encyclopaedia Britannica* describes the process of aging. It is part of the experience of living, as are infancy, childhood and adolescence.

A woman's body is typically in fullest bloom and in peak condition by her middle thirties, but it is already beginning to prepare for the cessation of its reproductive functions. Ovulation is occasionally skipped; previously regular menstrual periods may become a bit variable. A few women start the menopause process.

Yet today, more than in any previous time of history, many women in their mid- to late thirties are having a first baby. These are usually well-planned pregnancies, joyfully undertaken by secure and confident women who lead active lives and are in excellent health. Today's prenatal medical care, along with well-informed self-care, takes much of the risk out of first pregnancies in the mature years.

There are several theories about what causes those changes we identify as physical aging. One theory is that your lifespan is programmed in your genes, so when the preclocked time runs out, you'll stop living (provided, of course, that you exclude premature death from accident or disease). This theory may imply that aging signs as we know them are simply steps downward, toward an all-at-once loss of function. It's rather neat and rather fatalistic.

From what we know about human physiology, the various organs and tissues of our bodies are constructed to last much longer than the usual lifetime. So if the lifespan is indeed programmed in the genes, that clock is probably set for a life cycle of a couple of centuries or more—barring illness, injury, etc.

Another theory is that the body's molecules accumulate "errors" that eventually cause life's functions to stop. Signs of aging along the way represent errors in the messages between molecules, so that certain cells and organs fail to work properly. A similar concept holds that aging is the accumulation of mutated cells that are slightly changed as they grow and divide, so they don't perform normally and eventually bring about loss of organ function.

A simpler idea is the "wear and tear" theory, which holds that living creatures, like machines, just wear out. A problem with this notion is that unlike machines, we are biological beings and possess the marvelous power to rebuild and repair ourselves to a great degree.

We do know that aging brings on various kinds of tissue changes throughout the body, at differing rates in different people. Lean muscles diminish, a few cells at a time, leading to the shrunken look of age that we all know. Granules called lipofuscins are deposited in heart-muscle fibers—an aging process that actually begins before age twenty. A very gradual loss of elasticity takes place in skin, blood vessels and other tissues. This slight stiffening effect is attributed to the formation of "cross links" in molecules of collagen, the elastic protein of many body parts.

The good news is that proper health care, diet, exercise and rest can do wonders to defer the typical aging symptoms that are uncomfortable and inconvenient, such as stiffening muscles and joints. And even the signs of age in our appearance can be moderated, not to keep us looking twenty years old, but to make us our most attractive selves at forty, sixty, and eighty.

A look at some common effects of aging on specific body systems will give us some guidelines on how best to take care of ourselves and what routine medical attention we're likely to need as we grow older.

Bones and Teeth

Osteoporosis, a condition of thinning, brittle bones, is a threat to older women in particular. It is not a process of normal aging, but an age-associated disorder for which preventive means and treatment are available.

The bony skeleton is an organ, just like the stomach and the heart. Besides providing the structural frame that holds us up and permits us to move about, the bones serve as a storage and distribution facility. The manufacture of red blood cells occurs in bone marrow. Calcium, a mineral needed in every cell of the body and for multiple functions including brain and muscle activity, is stored in the skeleton, for which it provides hardness and strength, but when other body tissues call for calcium, the bones yield their supply—and keep on filling orders even to the point of depletion and fracture. This capability for "sacrifice" is one reason we look carefully at bones during the aging process; another reason is bone "turnover," or the skeleton's ability to add and remove materials to maintain itself and keep bones strong. When these two processes fail to balance, bone might build up abnormally or break down abnormally.

An abnormal loss of bone mineral, mainly calcium, produces osteoporosis. Bones become thin and brittle, and eventually fracture. Osteoporosis now accounts for an estimated 195,000 broken hips and 100,000 broken wrists every year in the United States. By far the greatest share of these accidents happens to older women. It is also estimated that some 31,500 people die of the complications of broken hips.

Researchers are trying to uncover the causes of osteoporosis and are exploring methods for treating and preventing the disorder. Aging alone is apparently not the cause, since some groups of people, notably black Americans, rarely have the condition, compared with white subjects of similar ages and bone densities.

Many physicians believe that a lack of estrogen is the underlying factor, for the incidence of osteoporosis is high among women past menopause and among women whose ovaries have been surgically removed—i.e., in both instances, estrogen is no longer secreted.

Fluoride, calcium, vitamin D and vitamin K in various combinations are being explored as treatments for osteoporosis, either to slow down or to stop bone loss. Estrogen replacement therapy is used traditionally and has been found successful in slowing down or stopping bone loss. Many doctors, however, do not prescribe long-term estrogen use because they believe it brings with it unacceptable risks of endometrial cancer. Others believe close monitoring and the use of an interrupted estrogen-dosage cycle, or the addition of progesterone, equalize the elements of risk and gain. (In Chapter 13 we will describe several recommendations for taking care of one's bones in mature life.)

Periodontal disease, or gum-line deterioration with possible loosening of teeth, is not a natural consequence of aging, though it's certainly prevalent in older people. Some authorities believe gum-line disease (called pyorrhea) is caused by invading bacteria. Others, including Leo Lutwak, M.D., Ph.D, of Akron General Hospital's Department of Medicine, believe the major dental problems of the elderly are related to osteoporosis. The demineralizing effect of osteoporosis starts with the jawbone, Dr. Lutwak points out. Teeth loosen as the bony sockets begin to lose their minerals. The slight movements of loosened teeth can damage gum tissues, which, in turn, get inflamed, recede and often expose tooth roots.

"Not all gum disease is related to bone loss," says Dr. Lutwak. "But when it is, it's my belief that loss of bone starts the gum disease, not the other way around." He's a firm believer in calcium supplementation. In one of his studies of jawbone deterioration, a full year of calcium supplementation at the rate of one gram daily succeeded in stopping the bone thinning and even restored some of the lost bone mass.

Like many other body conditions generally believed to be consequences of aging, the breakdown and loss of tooth and bone substances are definitely not parts of the natural aging process, authorities say. They are largely preventable, usually treatable, and sometimes they can be reversed.

Your Lungs

The normal process of aging presents very little threat to healthy lungs. For one thing, a pair of lungs has about 300 million alveoli, or tiny air sacs; more than enough even if a large number should cease to function. Lung capacity—that is, the amount of air you can take in—decreases somewhat as years go by, and the amount of air you can exhale also becomes slightly diminished with time. Then, too, the rib cage becomes a trifle stiffer, and chest muscles may not be as strong as they were in one's youth. But for all ordinary purposes, the touch of age is feather-light on the breathing apparatus. The real threats to respiratory health are smoking, other air pollutants, infections and allergies. The greatest of these is smoking, a habit that invites not only lung cancer and heart disease but also disabling, life-threatening lung diseases such as emphysema and chronic bronchitis.

Your Brain and Nerves

The threat of senility, with its forgetfulness, confusion and disorientation, is, to many people, the most fearful prospect of aging. In earlier years, doctors and patients alike assumed that a breakdown in mental functioning, when it happened, was simply an effect of advanced age. Not true. Senility is a disease condition; aging is not. There are literally scores of disorders that produce symptoms of brain impairment, many of them medically treatable. These days when an older person shows behavioral or psychological changes, the alert physician checks for a medical cause: a bump on the head, a fever, improper nutrition, a drug reaction or psychological depression.

It's true that the brain loses a few neurons, or nerve cells, each day —and this goes on in all of us, starting in early adulthood. But the loss is very slight, and considering the enormous number of brain cells we have, those that are lost amount to only a few grains of dust from a mountain of brain matter. Loss of brain *function*, however, is not a part of healthy old age. Where brain damage occurs, it may be from a disease condition which causes a reduction in oxygen supply.

Both scientific testing and human experience affirm that ongoing years bring a very gradual slowing of nerve reflexes and reaction times. Testing also shows that while younger people generally assimilate data faster, older persons are more likely to excel in organizing the data into concepts. Memory is indeed more of a problem as one grows older; judgment, on the other hand, may improve with age. A key to continuing good mental function, the experts say, is to keep up intellectual activity and study.

Your Heart and Blood Vessels

The heart is a powerful muscle, built to last a great deal longer than the rest of your body. Even though it gradually loses muscle fibers and collects granular deposits, the healthy heart continues to be more than capable of meeting the demands customarily placed upon it. It does undergo a very gradual decline in performance, and at age ninety it pumps less blood than in youth. Still, in response to exercise, the aged heart can triple its ordinary pumping capacity. The key is exercise. The evidence is that older people need regular physical activity even more than young people do.

Hardening of the arteries—arteriosclerosis—has long been associated with the aged and has been widely considered an inevitable consequence of the passing years. But that's not necessarily so. Arteriosclerosis is a disease that can affect young people as well as older ones. When and if it occurs, you would be wise to regard it as a medically treatable condition rather than becoming resigned to it as an infirmity.

The gradual loss of elasticity in the blood vessels can cause a progressive increase in blood pressure as one grows older. But again, this doesn't necessarily happen. In the United States and Europe, an increase in blood pressure with age is so common that many doctors regard it as normal. An example would be a woman whose blood-pressure level was 112/70 at age twenty and is 156/80 as she reaches her eightieth birthday. But a look at other population groups shows that rising blood pressure as life progresses is probably not "normal" but merely typical in industrialized countries at this time in history. (In Chapter 13 we will talk more about the management of blood pressure.)

Atherosclerosis, the build-up of fatty plaques inside your blood vessels, is not necessarily a condition of aging. There exists persuasive evidence, though not proof, that dietary habits can help prevent the clogging of arteries. There's also evidence that staying lean and active helps keep the proper cholesterol balance between high-density lipoproteins (HDLs) and low-density lipoproteins (LDLs). HDL, the cholesterol fraction that keeps blood-vessel walls cleared, should be present at high levels; LDL scores should be kept as low as possible. (See Chapter 13 for more details.)

Your Digestive System

There's no reason why growing older should, by itself, bring on impaired digestion or absorption, and usually it does not. Your digestive system, properly maintained and kept free of disease, should work beautifully throughout your whole life. There may be a very gradual, very slight decrease in the production of hydrochloric acid in the stomach, along with some other digestive enzymes. But the absorption of sugar, proteins, vitamins and minerals should be almost as good in advanced age as in youth. Some studies indicate that there's a mild decrease in fat absorption, and this might explain why persons in their eighties and nineties are usually—but not always—rather thin. (It may also mean that thin people are generally more likely to reach those ages.)

Although digestive problems are common among older people, the bright side is that they are generally not the inevitable consequence of aging and are treatable. With self-knowledge and self-care, many chronic digestive conditions are also *preventable.* In the next chapter we will discuss ways and means for maintaining good digestive function.

Your Eyes and Ears

Aging does affect your eyes. Beginning at about age ten, the crystalline lens of the eye undergoes a very gradual stiffening. The ability to focus on nearby objects decreases at the same slow pace—an infinitesimal pace when you consider that a number of people have very good eyesight when they reach a hundred. Eye specialists say that most persons past fifty have age-related far-sightedness, called presbyopia, which means quite literally "old eyes." Other eye conditions—cataracts, glaucoma, and macular degeneration—are not caused by aging, but they are more likely to develop during the mature years.

There's a very slow decrease in the size of the eye's pupil as one ages. Also, a tiny loss of cells gradually cuts one's ability to see in dim light. This means that older people may need brighter lighting and probably will benefit from stepped-up illumination in living and work quarters, for better vision and safety. Night blindness, another form of the inability to see in dim light, also may be associated with nutritional deficiencies, notably of vitamin A and zinc.

For ordinary purposes, an individual's ability to hear changes very little with advancing age. After age fifty there is some loss of very-high-frequency sounds (the high notes on a piano, for example), and few persons over age sixty-five can hear frequencies above 10,000 cycles per second. The evident prevalence of hearing problems among the elderly probably results from the fact that there has been a longer span of time for the difficulties to develop. Occupational exposure to excessive noise can, however, exact a toll in hearing loss; so can greatly amplified music. Exposure to noise or complications arising from viral infections can also cause the buzzing, ringing or crackling ear sounds known as tinnitus.

Your Reproductive Tract

While the heart, lungs, digestion and other body systems must continue to serve you throughout life, the reproductive system is, in effect, permitted to retire. And so the single most significant event of the climacteric, for most women, is menopause. Ovulation, and with it menstrual bleeding, comes to a gradual stop. Estrogen and other hormones that have acted together in cycles for thirty years or more now begin to dwindle. The whole body adjusts, to some extent. As ovaries supply smaller amounts of estrogen—which are still needed for body maintenance—adrenal glands may step in to supply androstanedione, which can be converted to estrogen. FSH levels rise.

So-called hot flashes are the most common, puzzling and disturbing symptom during the menopause process. The face reddens in a sudden blush, a burst of sweat covers the entire body, and minor heart palpitations occur. Also at this time, vaginal tissues may become dry and fragile, so that intercourse is difficult or painful. A long-range problem that affects some women is weakening of support tissues inside the pelvic area. This can lead to displacement of the bladder or uterus.

Psychological symptoms once commonly attributed to menopause are now being re-evaluated, and scientific investigators are concluding that "menopause blues" is a myth. It is, of course, possible to have emotional problems at this or any other time of life, but evidence supports the view that these are not related to the process of menopause. (We'll discuss this more fully in Chapter 13.)

Menopause doesn't happen all at once. Ovulation is very likely to skip, resume, stop for months, and then occur again, like the last few kernels of popping corn. When a woman asks, "Have I stopped ovulating?," she usually wants to know whether she can become pregnant. It's a difficult question for a physician to answer.

In the same woman, ovulatory events can go on for several years. In one typical case, a woman's periods definitely stopped. She began having occasional hot flashes. Blood tests showed that her FSH levels were high, and her urine estrogen levels were low. In short, she had all the common signs of menopause. But after several months she began menstruating again. At that time her FSH levels were low and urine estrogen rose—every indication of resumption of ovulation.

During such off-again-on-again times, the functioning of the pituitary gland (whose secretions act to regulate other glands) and ovaries, marching in step together these many years, may be off phase. The luteal phase, in which the corpus luteum secretes progesterone, may be shortened. The likelihood of pregnancy is quite low, not because of the absence of ovulation but because the hormonal sequence is out of sync. Nevertheless, pregnancy can occur, as many women who considered themselves menopausal have found. This situation can cause any of a number of problems, such as unwanted pregnancy, high-risk pregnancy or the alternative of staying on the pill.

Absence of menstrual flow in a woman near age forty doesn't necessarily mean that she's entering menopause. If she has recently stopped using the pill, it may be post-pill amenorrhea, which leaves the ovulation picture uncertain. It may mean pregnancy. Or the condition may signal an endocrine (glandular) disorder. In any event, it's a time for regular medical monitoring and guidance by a doctor expecting all to be well but remaining alert to the possibility of problems. A rule of thumb—not always the case—is that when menstrual periods are regular, ovulation is probably going on as usual. After two years with no menstrual periods, ovulation is unlikely but not impossible.

Growing enlightenment on health and aging has, in recent years, presented us the gift of a renewed lease on life. The most recent of the National Institutes of Health, the National Institute on Aging, supports research on the aging processes, the health factors of later years, and the ways in which age-related health problems can be overcome. The goal of this and other research is not merely to extend the human lifespan so that people can spend more years being "old," but rather to improve health and medical practices so that millions of us can remain young for many added years.

13

ACTIVE HEALTH IN THE CLIMACTERIC YEARS

Aging has no effect upon you as a person. When you are "old" you will feel no different and be no different from what you are now or were when you were young, except that more experiences will have happened. In old age your appearance will change, however, and you may encounter more physical problems. When you do, these will affect you only as physical problems affect a person of any age. An "aged" person is simply a person who has been there longer than a young person.

Your memory, sexuality, activity, capacity for relationships and zest should normally last as long as you do, and do last in the majority of people. When they do not, it is for the same cause as in earlier years, namely illness.

—*Alex Comfort,*
A Good Age

What's so different about the way in which a woman should take care of her health in mature years? The lifelong "ground rules for health" outlined in Chapter 2 are useful guides whatever one's age. But there are special health considerations that merit special attention by women in the climacteric, for the following reasons:

• Times have changed, and with them social attitudes toward aging have changed. Today's mature woman has every reason to expect to continue an active and vigorous life. Menopause no longer means retirement from sports, sexuality or the pursuit of exciting new interests.

• For most older women, their life pattern has changed from what it was in their younger years. Many are widowed or divorced. For many whose children have grown, the scene has changed from a large, busy family to a suddenly quiet, two-person or one-person household.

• The normal changes of aging call for special emphasis in certain aspects of health care.

In this chapter we will discuss general maintenance and care in some primary areas of life: diet, exercise, sexuality, work and medical care. In each, there are some considerations affecting mature women, some questions to ask ourselves, and some answers to be sought independently and individually.

Diet, Nutrition and Digestion

Eating wisely and well may be the most important thing you do for your health at any time of your life. Poor eating habits or dietary neglect in the mature years can be particularly dangerous and can lead to a descending spiral of impaired digestion, lack of appetite, and eventual breakdown of health, and may result in a woman who is always tired and has no pep.

The most prevalent dietary pitfalls for older people are on the one hand obesity, a greater threat to health than in your younger years, and on the other undernutrition from indifference and lack of interest in food, often a consequence of loneliness.

The need for essential nutrients, including vitamins, minerals and proteins, remains at about the same level from early adulthood throughout the remainder of your life. The need for some nutrients, such as calcium, may actually rise. But in your mature years, beginning at approximately the age of fifty, the metabolic rate decreases, and therefore the daily calorie requirement goes down. The National Research Council's *Recommended Dietary Allowances* calls for 200 fewer calories a day for the woman past fifty-one than for the woman between twenty-three and fifty. A woman in her fifties should consume only about two thirds of the calories she did at age fourteen.

Since it's important to keep ingesting vitamins and minerals while lowering the calories, the older woman needs to follow a more precisely controlled, carefully chosen diet than ever before. (See charts in Chapter 2.)

A first step can be taken quite simply: stay away from sweets such as candy and soft drinks, and fatty foods such as rich sauces and visible fat on meat. Don't eat the skin of poultry; it's mostly fat. Use restraint in cocktails, wine and beer, not only to avoid the detrimental effects of overindulgence but because drinks carry a load of "empty" calories that lack compensating nutritional value.

The use of complex carbohydrates, or starches, as a major source of calories in place of fats and simple carbohydrates such as sugars is recommended by many nutritionists. This program is easy to follow and involves eating more fiber-bearing foods: whole grains, rice and legumes (peas, beans and lentils); fresh fruit and vegetables are a must.

Fiber, or roughage, is simply indigestible material, and it is back in style since medical research linked high-fiber diets to a reduced incidence of stomach and colon cancer, heart disease, hemorrhoids, constipation and diverticulitis. After many years of progressively eliminating fiber from our foods by "refining" them, we've discovered the body really needs fiber. Older people who live alone too often subsist on canned or frozen "convenience" foods; they have a special need of dietary bulk in order to maintain good bowel function. Generous use of raw fruit, vegetables and whole grains is essential as well as infinitely more appetizing than a diet consisting largely of refined and processed foods. One easy way to ensure a basic amount of fiber in your daily diet is to use one or two tablespoons of plain bran in your breakfast cereal.

You should also not overlook the condition of your teeth. Bad teeth are a common source of poor digestion among older people. When teeth are missing or in need of repair, the chewing process becomes inadequate. When stomach upsets result, the person is likely to turn to soft foods. A soft diet is almost always inadequate in several vitamins and minerals, and lacks food fiber. At worst, it's a "there goes the neighborhood" situation: three important systems —dental, digestive and nutritional—become impaired together. The bottom line is to keep your teeth in good repair for the sake of your overall health.

Unwise use of laxatives, a common practice among older persons, takes a needless toll on health. In Chapter 4 we discussed the problems that cause and are caused by constipation affecting women of any age. If constipation has become chronic, or if it is prompted by a medical condition, you should seek medical help. Then, by all means follow the self-care rules your physician advises. Chronic use of laxatives can impair bowel function. The use of mineral oil as a laxative can set off various kinds of trouble. It can block vitamin absorption, and it can also cause oil, or lipid, pneumonia if it is regurgitated and drawn into the windpipe.

For the health and strength of your skeleton into advanced years, both good nutrition and exercise, or weight-bearing activity, are essential. Bone is not, as we have mentioned, static. Bone substance builds up and is discarded at a steady rate; trouble in the form of osteoporosis, or thinning bones, can occur when the rebuilding process is blocked or prevented. Insufficient calcium or the inability to incorporate calcium into bone tissue may take place when estrogen supplies fail. Robert P. Heaney, M.D., of Creighton University in Omaha, Nebraska, has concluded that women need 800 milligrams of calcium daily before menopause, and about 1,500 milligrams daily after menopause in order to prevent bone loss. Other nutrition experts also affirm that older women need much more calcium than they required in earlier years. If you obtain your calcium from milk alone, you would need to take about 1 1/3 quarts every day to ingest the amount of calcium Dr. Heaney recommends for the postmenopausal woman.

A complicating factor in calculating the amount of calcium needed for bone maintenance is the calcium-phosphorus ratio. Phosphorus, another mineral nutrient, combines with calcium to form bone. But in the functioning of the human system, phosphorus and calcium are needed in approximately equal amounts, and any excess of phosphorus will act to cancel out calcium. So we should keep in mind that many of our nutritionally valuable foods—meat, poultry, seafood—contain many times more phosphorus than calcium. This is why we need considerable amounts of foods containing more calcium than phosphorus. Green leafy vegetables have three to four times as much calcium as phosphorus; oranges and pineapples have twice as much; and milk has about one-quarter more calcium than phosphorus.

It's highly likely that a favorable calcium-to-phosphorus ratio accounts for the excellent bone condition of some people who are vegetarians. Studies made in England of ovolactovegetarians (who eat no meat but do eat eggs and dairy foods) showed almost twice the amount of bone tissue in them—indicating excellent rebuilding function—than in matched subjects who were meat eaters.

A diet pattern that not only limits the total caloric intake but also controls the proportion of total calories coming from fat is regarded, according to today's metabolic knowledge, as more healthful and probably protective against coronary heart disease. In the average American diet, more than 40 percent of the calories are derived from fatty sources. The American Heart Association recommends adjusting this so that no more than 35 percent of calories come from fat. In addition, saturated fatty acids, which are generally of animal origin, should amount to less than one third of total daily fat intake. But calories trimmed away from fatty food sources should not be made up in simple carbohydrates, or sugars. For some persons, this could increase the risk of raising blood triglycerides, another predisposing factor for heart trouble.

It's still a matter of scientific controversy whether restricting foods with a high-cholesterol content—eggs, for instance—helps to keep blood cholesterol within normal limits and helps to prevent the deposition of fatty plaques on blood-vessel walls. High blood cholesterol, or hyperlipidemia, is associated with increased rates of coronary heart disease. Since the body makes its own cholesterol, it has been argued that food cholesterol isn't necessarily carried directly into the bloodstream or deposited on blood-vessel walls. Two kinds of fatty proteins that have been identified appear to have opposite effects: HDL (high-density lipoprotein) seems to hinder aggregation of the disk-shaped blood cells called platelets inside blood vessels, thereby preventing clotting, while LDL (low-density lipoprotein) forces platelets to collect into clumps—the clotting action that stops bleeding. For purposes of heart protection, we need to keep HDL levels high and LDL levels low. In studies to date, some factors that tend to raise the HDL level include regular, vigorous activity; low total fat intake in food; the use of replacement estrogens; weight loss; and moderate use of alcohol. HDL levels appear to go up as one grows older. Factors that cause HDL to go down, depriving one of this protective element, include weight gain and cigarette smoking. Heart experts say that smoking causes platelets to become sticky, tending to clog the blood vessels. Shortage of the artery-clearing HDL can be the reason.

Researchers are now exploring the possibility that the consumption of fish, rather than meat, as a dietary fat source may help protect against platelet clumping inside blood vessels. Fatty acids known as EPA and ETA appear to protect Eskimos from atherosclerosis, despite their traditionally high-fat diet. Foods with high proportions of these protective fatty acids include scallops, oysters and red caviar.

Restraint in the use of salt may be of particular value for the older woman as her susceptibility to high blood pressure increases. Elderly persons who have gradual sensory losses in taste and smell may unconsciously increase salt in an effort to achieve flavor. It's a good idea to explore nonsalty condiments such as herbs and spices, and lemon and lime juice.

Exercise: Take a Piece of the Action

A test group of people who exercised vigorously over a ten-year haul had, according to nutrition authority Jean Mayer, Ph.D., 64 percent fewer heart attacks than their counterparts who were inactive. Exercise also confers many other benefits, such as improved muscle tone and a decidedly better appearance and figure control. Best of all is the inner sense of well-being and a frank, zesty approach to living. Exercisers feel better, and they know it.

The information and guidelines on exercise for women as given in Chapter 2 also applies to women in their mature years. One simply gears one's activity to individual capabilities, as always.

In Chapter 2, it was noted that cross-country skiing and handball or squash can burn up satisfying amounts of energy as calories. Dr. Mayer has published a list of calorie expenditures for other activities. The following calorie usages are based on 1 hour of action:

Canoeing: At 2.5 miles per hour, 180 calories. At 4 miles per hour, 420.
Climbing: 700 to 900 calories.

Cycling: At 5 miles per hour, 250 calories. At 10 miles per hour, 450. At 14 miles per hour, 700.

Dancing: According to Dr. Mayer, 200 to 400 calories. Almost certainly more calories for disco dancing.

Horseback: Walking, 150; trotting, 500; galloping, 600 (though even the horse is unlikely to gallop for an hour).

Golfing: 300 calories.

Gymnastics: 200 to 500 calories.

Rowing: At peak effort, 1,200 calories.

Running: 800 to 1,000 calories.

Sculling: At 20 strokes per minute, 420 calories. At 37 strokes per minute, 370.

Soccer: 550 calories.

Squash: 600 to 700 calories.

Sitting (at rest): 15 calories.

Skiing: 600 to 700 calories.

Standing (relaxed): 20 calories.

Swimming: Breast and backstroke, 300 to 650 calories. Crawl, 700 to 900.

Walking: Slow, about 2.5 miles per hour, 115 calories. Moderate, 3.75 miles per hour, 215. Very fast, 5.5 miles per hour, 565.

Writing: 20 calories.

If you are unaccustomed to regular exercise and decide to get started, it's wise to:

• Get a good physical checkup from your doctor, who can tell you whether you have any limitations that should be taken into account. The examination may include an electrocardiogram and a treadmill or step-test.

• Always warm up before starting a strenuous activity such as a tennis game.

• If you have a health impairment, such as a cardiac or chronic lung condition, you nonetheless need exercise. Ask your physician to prepare an exercise program for you, or he can refer you to a therapist or trainer who will give you a program designed for your needs.

Sex and Romance

> In the future, sex in the late years will be taken for
> granted. Then we will see for the first time the full life
> cycle of love and sexuality, with youth a time for
> exciting exploration and self-discovery; middle age for
> gaining skill, confidence and discrimination, and old
> age for bringing the experience of a lifetime, and the
> unique perspectives of the final years to the art of
> loving one another.
>
> —Robert Butler, M.D., director,
> National Institute on Aging

The misconception that older persons are not normally interested in, or capable of, sexual intercourse is fortunately fading out. Yet the fact that desire and desirability in older men and women are not past attainment nor unseemly still needs to be stressed.

Misconceptions about the sexuality of older people can probably be traced to the nineteenth-century view that women normally had no sexual feelings. In more recent times many doctors simply did not consider the possibility of ongoing sexuality. Now virtually all physicians are aware that older people can of course be sexually active. "The figures . . . show that older people are and always have been sexually active, but that they are getting less embarrassed about it as the culture gets less uptight about sexuality generally," writes Alex Comfort, M.D., in his book *A Good Age.*

What are the actual physical facts of aging and sexuality, excluding those that are psychologically self-imposed and dispelling those that are based on faulty notions from folklore and tradition?

A major change caused by aging is that orgasm may occur less frequently, and that the man may need longer stimulation to produce an erection. Some female partners welcome this, since it means more leisurely, sensuous love-making. Sometimes the male erection fails, simply from fatigue, that extra drink or two, or some outside stress or worry. Some men can become so frightened by one failure that the problem becomes compounded—another penalty of the old, erroneous idea that aging spells impotence for men. Says Dr. Butler: "All men of any age are impotent from time to time." But in the absence of disease—and even some conditions once sexually disabling are now responding to treatment—sexual needs and capabilities can be lifelong for both men and women who wish them to continue, and who have or can find partners.

Clinical research is now achieving significant advances in understanding and overcoming male impotence, with much of the gain in the area of improved and more accurate diagnosis. Formerly, impotence was considered almost exclusively caused by psychological or emotional factors, with as few as 5 or 10 percent of the cases due to endocrine, or glandular, causes. Yet even with psychological therapy, failure rates were high—and those who failed to improve sadly accepted the idea that their mental and emotional blocks were insurmountable. A research team at Harvard Medical School found that more than one third of one patient group with impotence symptoms actually had unsuspected medical disorders, which were revealed by tests of male hormones in the blood. Most of these patients were successfully treated and had their potency restored.

On the other hand, a leading medical cause of impotence, diabetes, has been carefully reviewed in European tests. Men who were believed permanently impotent due to their diabetic condition were monitored during sleep. The cyclic erectile response that normally takes place in sleep was still happening in a significant number of these patients—again indicating that with appropriate treatment, potency might return.

The gynecologic problem of dyspareunia, difficult or painful intercourse, commonly arises in the later years as a result of estrogen shortages. Without sufficient estrogen, vaginal tissues may shrink and become thin, fragile and dry. Estrogen replacement therapy, when medically advisable, may take care of this problem. Researchers have lately found that vaginal estrogen creams and lotions can raise the estrogen level of the blood just as pills do. In these cases, non-estrogen lubricating creams can be very helpful. These can be prescribed or can be purchased at drugstore counters. Be sure to use only those products specifically intended as vaginal moisturizers or lubricants.

Some conditions that may affect sexuality—and older people more often than younger ones—are these:

- *Heart disease.* Some men and women give up sexual intercourse once they've had a heart attack, usually because they're afraid it will set off another attack. The incidence of heart attacks during coitus is, however, thought to be very low; and intercourse is believed to be no more responsible for coronary disease than sleeping, running or eating, or any other normal activity.

The major problem is resuming sexual intercourse following the necessary sexual abstinence during recovery. Dr. Butler says that sexual activity can, and usually should, be resumed about sixteen weeks after a heart attack, depending on one's physical condition. Resumption should be planned and thoroughly discussed with the physician, both for guidance and for the reassurance of both partners. A test of readiness, according to Dr. Butler, is the ability for one to walk vigorously for three blocks or climb one or two flights of stairs without pain or adverse changes in pulse, blood pressure or electrocardiogram readings.

• *Anemia.* This is a common and generally easily treated condition; it is said to affect one out of four people past sixty years of age. Anemia causes fatigue, the natural enemy of sexual activity. Often nutritional correction, with an improved diet and added vitamins and minerals, will correct the anemic condition and restore bodily energy and sexual vigor at the same time.

• *Drugs.* Prescribed medications, including tranquilizers, antidepressants and some high-blood-pressure drugs, can cause loss of sexual function. If this should happen to you or your mate, the problem should by all means be discussed with your physician. Often the doctor can either adjust the dosage or change the prescription to a less inhibiting drug. But the doctor must be informed that the problem exists and that it is important to the patient.

• *Alcohol.* Drinking is said to be the most widespread source of sexual problems related to drugs—for alcohol is a drug. As any man knows who has ever had one drink too many, alcohol may stimulate arousal, but it also brings on temporary impotence—at any age. Excess alcohol reduces male potency and also delays orgasm in women. For older persons, a general rule of thumb—or elbow—is: No more than 1 1/2 ounces of hard liquor *or* two 6-ounce glasses of wine *or* three 8-ounce glasses of beer in any 24-hour period when sexual activity is anticipated.

• *Emotional problems.* While the essence of romance is emotion,

and the mysterious and unmeasured psyche underlies all great experiences including love, the realm of feeling is also most often the
place where loss of function begins. Men who are alarmed by a slight
and gradual slowing of their sexual responses can stampede themselves into real impotence. Women who see in themselves the signs
of maturity replacing the provocative sexiness of youth often start
worrying about whether it's proper for them to engage in love play.
This is most likely a hangup straight out of yesteryear, when many
of us, as girls, received the strong impression that nice old ladies—
anybody past the age of thirty—were through with sex. In films and
advertising, romance and passionate love have generally been por-
trayed only by young persons, and until quite recently, sexual interest on the part of middle-aged or older couples was considered
comic or improper. But May-December romance, as in *South Pacific,*
was quite all right as long as the female lead represented May, or
youth. The sensible outlook is to recognize these stereotypes for
what they are, and heed only the real you. Older women are an
astonishingly diverse group of individuals, not society's role models.

In their book, *Love and Sex after Sixty,* Dr. Butler and his psycho-
therapist wife, Myrna Lewis, stress that it's not essential for all
elderly persons to feel compelled to have an interest in sex. But those
who *are* interested, the authors say, should not have to face restric-
tions. Drs. Butler and Lewis welcome the fact that some nursing
homes are arranging "privacy rooms" for couples to be alone together. "In the normal course of aging," says Dr. Butler, "women
ordinarily do not lose their physical capacity for orgasm, nor men
their capacity for erection and ejaculation. A pattern of regular
sexual activity, or at least self-stimulation, helps to preserve sexual
functioning in both men and women."

Shortage of male partners is a very real problem for older women.
To some extent the problem is numerical. According to statistics,
men die somewhat earlier than women. But much of the problem
is, once more, rooted in the traditions of society. Wives tend to be
younger than husbands, and therefore more likely to face widow-
hood in later life. It has been socially acceptable for older men to pair
off with much younger women, but not the other way around.
Today there is an increasing number of older women who are

forming bonds, including marriage, with younger men—just as older men have done all along with younger women.

The Butler-Lewis team finds still other trends that reflect our permissive society and create more sexual options for older women. Sexual fantasy, masturbation and sexual massage, for example, are among these alternatives. Physical attachments between women are also more widely accepted than in past times. Of course, many people find some of these options unacceptable on religious or moral grounds.

It seems clear that the sexual problems of older people are not much different in kind, only in certain aspects, from those of younger persons. Along with other concerned specialists, Dr. Butler urges older people to communicate their sexual concerns to their doctors and if necessary to request referral to a qualified sex therapist.

Work

This is a society traditionally based on work. Your work is a principal part of your identity, so that to most other people "you are what you do." This is generally true for both men and women, and at all economic, educational and social levels. Like everyone else, most women face a definite change in the kind of work they do at some point in their mature lives. The rearing of children comes to an end; office employment leads toward retirement; and factory work certainly does so.

At this juncture in their lives, women face a dilemma very much like the one they probably encountered back in their late teens or early twenties: What shall I become? What role or type of work is best for me? *What am I going to be when I grow up?* For nothing less than a second growing-up is at hand, whether it involves retirement, a new career or a new pattern of home life. It's important to your health and well-being—and of course may be important to your livelihood—to make occupational plans for the mature years. On this second round of pathfinding, the options may be wider than you realize.

The people who look forward with enthusiasm to "retiring" are those with plans and prospects for a new activity: building a dream house; raising a garden, or horses, or dogs; starting a new business; "catching up" on travel, or painting, or writing or taking college courses.

Support Groups

It's easy enough to say that the continuation of useful activity into the mature years is essential to every woman's health, well-being and self-esteem, but for many women this turning point can pose enormous problems. A woman faces such questions as to whether to continue with her accustomed type of employment or to move into a new phase of experience by learning a new job. Or if a woman has not previously had a regular job, she may face the need to find paid employment or be obliged to establish a new living pattern. Meeting new challenges such as these can be frightening for the woman who doesn't have the requisite background or who has some physical limitation or who has lived a private life, out of the social or occupational mainstream.

Deep-rooted prejudices still prevail toward older people in business, industry and society as a whole. Reduced spending power is a major problem with older people, especially those on a fixed income now riddled by inflation. And the winds of politics, as reflected in employment, housing, education and taxes, have threatened at times to push older Americans right out of their well-earned places in business, industry and community life.

Prospects for fairer treatment are improving. Many employers prefer older women in certain types of jobs because of their competence, stability, courtesy and dignity in meeting the public.

Only in recent years have older men and women recognized their political force. People past sixty-five now make up America's fastest-growing age group. In 1980 they numbered 24 million—11 percent of the population—and they will reach 32 million by the year 2000. Any group of such size, particularly one bound together by common interests, carries political power that can lead to improvement in public policy and recognition of the health, housing, education, employment and other needs of its members.

• Each of the fifty states now has an Office on Aging, funded by the federal government under the Older Americans Act. These are linked to six hundred area agencies on aging, and over a thousand senior citizen centers. Government-backed projects can provide help in the forms of services, information and activities for persons age fifty-five and older. Look in the telephone book under city or state government listings; people at these offices can direct you to programs that include health, exercise, nutrition, food purchase, employment, housing, taxes, legal assistance and medical care. Remember that these services are in no sense charity; they are facilities your taxes have helped to fund, and you are fully entitled to participate in their benefits.

• Community women's centers generally serve women of all age groups; they often operate food cooperatives, services to the disabled, family counseling, sales outlets for clothing and handmade goods, and have club interests of various kinds. In mature years, women who have been fully occupied with family or career may find for the first time that women's organizations offer much-needed help as well as rewarding activities. And you can give help as well as get it.

• Women's networks—a new term and a renewed concept— amount to a concerted but decentralized movement of women helping one another. In their quest for opportunities equal to those of men, a few women leaders began to assess the power of "old-boy networks," the loyalties that influence a corporate executive, for example, to employ or promote another male who went to his prep school or college, who belongs to his club or who moves in his social set. As women saw it, preferential treatment and advancement for men often began in men's luncheon clubs, bars and locker rooms— in all-male social situations. Women's roles in such networks appeared to be secondary, as wives, daughters or social subordinates.

Deciding that male networks were a strong enough force to exclude women from job and professional opportunities, women have set to work forming and strengthening their own network ties. The basic groups take up diverse interests. There are music networks, sports networks, professional networks such as groups of women physicians and lawyers, support groups such as rape crisis centers and havens for battered wives. And there are also organizations that focus on the problems, as well as the growing opportunities, of older women. The network idea means, of course, that these organizations get in touch with one another, offer one another help and information when needed, and foster countless one-to-one acquaintanceships between women—very much like an extended community of neighbors.

Medical Care

Managing your medical care, like the management of your diet, exercise and living habits, becomes ever more a fine art as you grow older. Some medical considerations apply more strongly to older women than to younger ones, and increasingly so into advanced age.

Paula B. Goldberg, Ph.D., assistant professor of pharmacology at the Medical College of Pennsylvania, whose special interest is drug response in the aging process, provides some useful guidelines toward managing medications wisely:

• Resist building up a whole array of frequently used medicines, either prescribed or over-the-counter purchases. It has been reported that elderly persons take, on the average, 5.6 prescription and nonprescription drugs at the same time—at great risk of drug interactions that may either cancel or increase the effect of a medicine.

• Never take prescription drugs left from an earlier illness. A current illness may be quite different from an earlier one, even when the symptoms are similar. Also, you may have forgotten why the drug was first prescribed and resume taking it for the wrong purpose. Or the medicine may have deteriorated chemically.

• Don't borrow or trade medications; it is dangerous to take someone else's medicine even if your ailment seems similar to the one the other person has.

• If you forget to take a dose of a prescribed medicine, or if you are going to bed early, don't double up on the dosage unless your doctor advises it. A missed dose is usually less dangerous than a double dose.

• Aspirin can cause stomach irritation, especially in older persons. Coffee and alcoholic drinks may increase this effect. If you take aspirin, be sure to drink generous amounts of fluid, preferably milk, to buffer the irritation. If you take drugs for ulcers, gout, diabetes or other disorders, don't take aspirin without consulting your doctor. People with bleeding disorders, those on anticoagulants or those scheduled for surgery should not take aspirin.

• Medicines other than aspirin have also heightened effects when mixed with alcohol or caffeine. Be sure your physician knows whether you drink beer, wine, whiskey, coffee, tea or cola. Also tell him about your smoking habits.

• Laxatives and antidiuretic drugs can change your absorption of drugs; if you're on prescribed medication, don't use these drugs without consulting your doctor.

• Be cautious about using antacid preparations. Seltzers contain large amounts of sodium, which can be dangerous to people on salt-restricted diets, those using diuretics or those who are taking drugs for heart disorders. Antacids can also mask stomach-ulcer symptoms. If you have indigestion more than once every two weeks, or if it's associated with shortness of breath or vomiting, see your doctor.

14

CANCER

You have cancer. Or your mother or sister does. The first rule is, don't panic at the mere mention of the word. Fortunately, many types of cancer, particularly gynecologic cancers, are completely curable. Most gynecologic oncologists (cancer specialists) go on giving periodic checkups to a large number of women who have been successfully treated for their early cancers and who are living perfectly ordinary lives.

If you or a loved one has a type of cancer you have reason to believe is not curable, don't give up hope for a long and productive life, possibly made even more precious by the daily awareness of how fragile life really is. People who know they have cancer do not live a life different in substance from everyone else; they merely live with a heightened consciousness of the fact that all of us have been allotted only a finite time to survive.

Facing the diagnosis is difficult. Initially there is a stage when the woman fears she is being protected from the worst of the news, and it is true that many physicians hesitate to lay heavy-handed pronouncements on a patient. Many people really do prefer to remain in ignorance; but for the patient who wishes to "know all," direct, open questions to her physician will usually indicate her willingness and ability to deal with her affliction. It is often wise to include a family member or a close friend in discussions with the physician; a third person may later be able to recall the details more accurately and be helpful in sharing the natural grieving process with the patient.

Most women benefit from an honest discussion of the medical findings and the prognosis (which means the doctor's estimate of what lies ahead). The patient who can cope with the reality or fact establishes a bond of honesty between herself and her physician that allows her to air her concerns; one who cannot cope with the reality quickly enlists psychological defenses of denial and amnesia to block out what was said, thus providing the physician with valuable clues as to how much the patient will be able to "take" in the future.

It is difficult to accept a grim, merciless prognosis. There is something in the human soul that refuses to give up hope. Many will grab at straws—citing reports of "miracle vitamins" or "wonder drugs" that promise a cure. There is no assurance that a chemotherapy regimen will be any more effective than a vitamin combination or a "wonder drug"; indeed, it is entirely possible that a vitamin or lack of one will inhibit the growth of tumor cells. But the drug treatments used by the medical community differ from those often touted through hearsay or magazine articles in that they have undergone extensive human and animal testing and are reviewed for effectiveness in controlled studies.

Perspective on life changes a great deal in a person who has cancer. When we're young and healthy, many of us express such sentiments as "If I get cancer, I'll get myself to a desert island with a good book and a bottle of booze," or "If you're dying of cancer, what's the difference between six months of survival and dying tomorrow?"

However, when we are really faced with the disease, the questions are more logical: Do you want to accept the dying process or do you want to try whatever may help cure you? Do you want to die next week or two months from now—after your daughter has graduated or your son married; after you have had time to make peace with your alienated sister? When truly faced with a short time to live, most of us will choose to undergo treatment that offers hope and a chance for those few extra months or years, during which every day can be treated as a special gift.

Coping with cancer, however, does not produce miracles in human interaction. Medical bills and the constant strain of living with the knowledge of cancer may intensify family conflicts. A heavy burden of guilt and fear is often laid on top of existing family problems: the daughter who has previously been rebellious and resentful now feels guilty about the pain she has caused her mother; yet the demands of a sick mother may make her even more resentful and angry. Families of the cancer patient—or any person with a chronic illness—must accept the fact that the worry, grief, anger at, resentment of, and still love and concern for the sick one can be a very trying mixture. Recognizing and accepting these feelings as normal parts of any human relationship and as normal ways of coping with illness can go a long way toward alleviating the pain they can cause.

If you do *not* have cancer, now is the time to be thinking about prevention and early-detection measures. If you smoke, stop. If it has been a long time since your last Pap smear, get one. If you do not do monthly breast exams on yourself, start. If you notice blood in your urine, have a chronic cough or any ongoing aches, pains or bleeding that have not been evaluated medically, have them checked out. Don't be like the woman who had vaginal spotting for two years before she went to see her physician—because she was "afraid I might have cancer." She did, and by then it was advanced cancer.

Cervical Cancer

Cervical cancer accounts for 11 percent of all cancers. It is second to breast cancer as the most common female malignancy, but represents about 50 percent or more of reproductive-tract tumors in women. About two out of 100 women develop cervical cancer each year, and some 10,000 women die from it annually. Although the above figures show a *relative* decrease in the proportion of cervical cancers compared to other female tumors, the incidence is actually not changing very much.

The good news is that with regular Pap smears, this disease can usually be picked up in the very early stages and can be cured. The bad news is that with increasing early and multipartner sexual activity, we can expect the incidence of cervical cancer to increase.

Many "risk factors" are associated with cervical cancer: early age of intercourse, sexual promiscuity, frequent and early childbearing, herpesvirus infections and uncircumcised male partners. Cervical cancer is almost unheard of in nuns. It is less common in Jewish women (possibly due to the effects of circumcision of all Jewish males), and twice as common in black women as in Caucasian females. In the Fiji Islands, cervical cancer is eight times more common in wives of uncircumcised males than in those women whose husbands are circumcised. There is, however, no good evidence that in populations with good hygenic practices that circumcision or lack thereof relate to the risk of cervical cancer. Women with herpesvirus infections are more likely to develop cervical cancer than noninfected women; women who have cervical cancer are more likely to have herpesvirus than control subjects do.

The exact reason for the above observations and the exact cause of cervical cancer are not known. It is felt that herpes or possibly some carcinogenic substance in the male smegma (penile discharge) may directly cause cervical cancer, which would account for a higher incidence in sexually promiscuous women, women with herpes infections, and women with uncircumcised partners. It is also felt that chronic irritation and scarring of the cervix may trigger the surface cells, the epithelium, into abnormal growth—hence the association with more births and chronic cervical infections. Racial and ethnic differences probably result from varying cultural and socioeconomic differences.

Cervical cancer, like most tumors, has various "stages," or extent of disease. There seems to be a slow progression from dysplasia (abnormal surface tissue) to carcinoma in situ (i.e., localized) to advanced cancer, although there is now some feeling that dysplasias may correct themselves spontaneously and may not necessarily progress. Any abnormal Pap smear, however, needs to be carefully followed up.

Stage I. The cancer is entirely confined to the cervix (may extend into the uterus and still be stage I). It is generally treated with hysterectomy, either simple hysterectomy for "microinvasive," or very early lesions, or a more extensive, or "radical," hysterectomy, which involves taking out a wide margin of vaginal and parametrial tissues (around uterus) if there is concern that the lesion may be seeding into a wider area (shedding cancer cells). An alternative treatment is radiation therapy by a trained therapist. There may be reasons in an individual case for doing either type of therapy or both, as well as for searching for lymph-node involvement. Prior to hysterectomy, the cervix must be carefully evaluated for the extent of disease. This may be done either by cone biopsy or colposcopically directed biopsy. (See Chapter 10 for detailed discussions of these techniques.)

Stage II. The tumor extends downward into the upper third of the vagina or area around the cervix but not to the pelvic side walls. Again, surgery (almost always radical hysterectomy) or radiation therapy may be used.

Stage III. The tumor is well down into the vaginal (IIIa) or pelvic sidewalls (IIIb) or there is evidence on x-ray of obstruction of the ureters (the tubes from kidneys to bladder). Occasionally very radical surgery can remove all of these tumors, but generally they are treated with radiation and can only rarely be cured. Chemotherapy may be employed when surgical therapy is impossible and radiation has already been tried.

Stage IV. The tumor has invaded the bladder or rectum (IVa) or has extended outside the pelvis (IVb). Palliative surgery, radiation therapy or chemotherapy may be employed; diversion of urine or stool through abdominal stomas (surgically constructed openings) may be necessary.

Endometrial Cancer

Since the recent publicity about a possible link between estrogen hormone use and carcinoma of the mucus membrane lining the uterus, this disease has received a great deal more attention. The good effects of this are that women are much more conscious of the necessity of seeking medical attention for any abnormal bleeding and that women consumers are looking with a healthy suspicion on hormonal therapy. Physicians are more careful about screening for endometrial cancer and very cautious about prescribing hormonal therapy. The bad effects are that the potential benefits of estrogen therapy may be neglected in the paranoia about any use of estrogens, in any dose or form, at any time.

Several other risk factors have been identified for endometrial cancer: obesity, low fertility, diabetes, hypertension, estrogen-secreting tumors, a history of abnormal uterine bleeding and late, gradual menopause. Endometrial cancer generally occurs in perimenopausal (around menopause) or postmenopausal women.

Endometrial cancer may be, but is not reliably, detected by a Pap smear. Many physicians are starting to do endometrial aspirates (sucking out some endometrial cells) in an office procedure, as a screening test for endometrial cancer. If you are concerned or feel you may be at risk for this disease, ask your physician about the possibility of an outpatient screening procedure. If you have any symptoms of abnormal bleeding, many physicians will prefer to do a D&C to be certain they get a very thorough sampling of endometrial and endocervical tissue. Any episode of postmenopausal bleeding (PMB) needs evaluation by a physician for possible cervical, endometrial or even ovarian causes. PMB is usually the first symptom and occurs early in endometrial cancer. Heavy or irregular bleeding in women nearing the menopause should also be evaluated. In fact, in *any* age group, abnormal bleeding should be evaluated by a physician, although most abnormal bleeding is *not* caused by cancer.

Endometrial cancers also have stages:

Endometrial hyperplasia. This is an excess growth of the endometrial tissue; some consider it a premalignant lesion. Occasionally progesterone therapy will make a hyperplastic endometrium return to normal, but any woman receiving progesterone for this condition must have very careful follow-up with D&Cs or endometrial biopsies to be sure no cancer develops in the endometrium. Sometimes endometrial hyperplasia requires a hysterectomy.

Stage 0. Carcinoma in situ is localized lesion. Many physicians recommend hysterectomy for this condition.

Stage I. The tumor is confined to the fundus (top of the uterus). Surgery often results in a complete cure, although radiation may be an alternative or additional means of therapy.

Stage II. The tumor has invaded the body of the uterus and the cervix. Again, this requires surgery. Radiation is often used in addition to surgery.

Stage III. The cancer has spread beyond the uterus but is not outside the pelvis. Surgery may or may not be feasible; radiation with or without chemotherapy is almost always recommended.

Stage IV. The tumor is outside the pelvis or invading the bowel or bladder. Palliative surgery or radiation may be helpful; chemotherapy may slow the spread of the tumor.

Ovarian Cancer

Ovarian cancer is increasing in frequency and, sadly, no reliable early-detection method yet exists. Many ovarian cancers do not give symptoms until they are widespread. Typically, an ovarian tumor will "seed" into the abdominal cavity, and only then does it cause symptoms. The woman will seek medical attention either because of the tumor's bulk or because it has begun to interfere with other organ systems.

The relative incidence of ovarian cancer is increasing perhaps in part due to the lack of early-detection methods. Among all the carcinomas in women, ovarian cancer is the fourth leading cause of death, exceeded only by cancer of the breast, colon and lung. (Although cervical cancer is more common, ovarian cancer is more likely to be fatal.)

The picture is not entirely bleak. A substantial proportion of ovarian "neoplasms," or growths, are relatively benign, with good prognoses. (See Chapter 11 for a discussion of dermoid tumors and ovarian cysts, conditions that are generally benign and affect young women.) Even with more advanced cancers some women do very well, particularly since the advent of chemotherapy treatments which have resulted in good remissions (lengthened freedom from disease) for a large number of women.

Ovarian cancer is a composite term for many different varieties of cancer. Since the ovary is created out of a number of different kinds of cells, tumors of the ovary are a complex grab bag of different types that may behave differently and have different prognoses.

In ovarian cancer, as in most other cancers, the "stage," or extent of disease, relates to the prognosis. Stage I disease is confined to the ovaries, and surgery is often curative. Stage II disease extends into the pelvis. Stage III has spread into the abdomen; stage IV has spread to the lungs or other organs outside the abdomen. Stages III and IV usually require radiation and/or chemotherapy in addition to surgery.

The symptoms of ovarian cancer vary, but one gynecologic text cites the following as "presenting symptoms": Abdominal swelling, 70 percent; abdominal discomfort, 50 percent; gastrointestinal difficulties (nausea, vomiting or diarrhea), 20 percent; urinary symptoms (frequency or urgency), 15 percent; abnormal bleeding, 15 percent; and weight loss, 15 percent. Nonsymptomatic ovarian cancer has a tendency to cause fluid accumulation in the abdomen called ascites. While in practice ovarian cancer is only rarely discovered as an ovarian mass on pelvic exam, any ovarian mass must be considered a serious finding and evaluated as a possible tumor. In a young woman the likelihood that an ovarian mass is a functional cyst (see Chapter 11) may prompt a physician to observe it over a period of a few weeks, but in general, ovarian masses require an operation. Any ovarian mass in a prepubertal girl or a postmenopausal woman should be considered an ovarian cancer until proven otherwise. Approximately 25 percent of established ovarian cancer patients will also have an abnormal Pap smear.

In general, treatment for ovarian cancer consists of total abdominal hysterectomy and bilateral salpingo-oophorectomy (removal of uterus, Fallopian tubes and both ovaries), along with removal of part of the omentum (fatty padding of the abdominal cavity), study of the cells in the peritoneal fluid, and thorough examination or biopsies at the time of surgery of all of the tissues in the abdominal cavity. Very occasionally, if a tumor is of a type considered to be fairly benign and if the patient is young with no children, the surgeon may remove only the tumor and leave the uterus and the opposite ovary intact. Often chemotherapy will be recommended following removal of an ovarian tumor, and sometimes radiotherapy is also recommended. If a woman responds very well to treatment and shows no further evidence of disease on chemotherapy, some medical centers advocate a "second look" operation to see if the patient is indeed free of the disease and if chemotherapy can be discontinued.

Less Common Genital Tumors

Although the malignancies listed below are rare, they should be mentioned briefly.

Vulvar cancer. Cancer of the vulva represents only one percent of all cancers in women, although recent reports indicate that it may be on the increase for reasons yet unknown. It tends to be a disease of elderly women (average age for invasive vulvar cancer is sixty-two years), but it can affect women of any age. The rule of thumb for detection of vulvar cancer is that anything on the vulva that looks abnormal needs medical attention. Treatment generally involves surgery with or without radiation therapy. The prognosis for early lesions is generally good; that for extensive tumors is poor.

Vaginal cancer. This condition is extremely rare. It generally represents the spread of a tumor from another organ. One specialized type has been found in young women whose mothers received DES during their pregnancy. (See Chapter 6.)

Uterine sarcomas. Sarcomas are a different cell line from carcinomas, but also can occur in the female genital tract. Uterine sarcomas may arise in fibroids, although very few (less than one percent) of fibroids turn out to be malignant. Generally, these tumors spread quickly and widely, although a few patients respond very well to treatment. Treatment may consist of surgery and radiation and may include chemotherapy.

Fallopian tube cancer. This is very rare and is generally detected only after it has spread.

Cancers of Other Systems

Except for breast cancer, which will be covered in some detail, it is not our purpose to go into detail on all possible cancers, but we do want to call your attention to warning signs of other types of cancers in the hope of getting you to your physician promptly should any of these signals arise.

Bladder cancer or renal (kidney) cancer. Often the first sign is painless but bloody voiding. Many benign conditions, such as infection, can also cause bloody urine, but any time you see blood in your urine, it is time for a checkup.

Colon and rectal cancer. The most common first symptom of these cancers is rectal bleeding or a change in type or caliber (i.e., thinning) of stool. Unless you are quite sure that a spot of blood is from a hard stool or a hemorrhoid, have it checked.

Skin cancer. Any skin sore that does not heal or any darkened area that seems to be new or enlarging needs to be examined and possibly biopsied. If you ever had skin x-ray treatment (it was a common treatment for acne at one time), or if you have had a lot of exposure to the sun, or if you smoke, you are at increased risk.

Lung cancer. This is less common in people who do not smoke or have not been occupationally exposed to dusts, such as coal or asbestos, known to cause lung cancer. Often this cancer is symptomless, but any chronic cough or coughing that brings up blood needs to be checked out. Of course, not every cough or even every bloody sputum is due to lung cancer!

Breast Cancer

Few diseases carry the terror for women that breast cancer does. The most common of female tumors, breast cancers comprise 25 percent of all female malignancies. Five out of every 100 women will at some time develop breast cancer, and half of the women with breast cancer will die from the disease. When you consider further that the treatments commonly employed are disfiguring, and that the disease attacks a part of the body that is extremely important emotionally and psychologically in our culture, then the common dread of breast cancer is indeed a logical response to a very grim situation.

First, however, a word of optimism: most breast masses, particularly in young women, are not malignant. Cystic disease, fibroadenomas and papillomas, as well as infections, can cause breast masses that are not malignant. So although any hard, new nodule noted in the breast should promptly be called to the attention of a physician and probably biopsied, many such masses will turn out to be benign conditions.

In general, the earlier breast cancer is found, the more likely it is to respond well to treatment. Women who examine themselves regularly and find a lump are the most likely to find them at an early stage. This is why all women should learn how to do breast self-examinations, and do them once a month. The best time is a day or two following a menstrual period, since just before menses the glandular development of breast tissue may feel nodular. After a

SELF-BREAST EXAMINATION

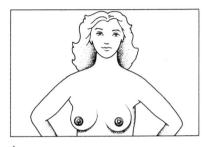

1.
Look at your breasts in the mirror for any irregularities or dimpling.

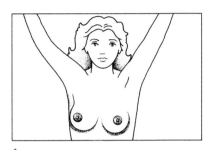

2.
Look again with your arms raised in the air.

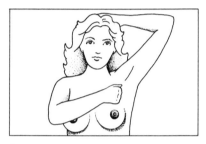

3.
Feel all around your breasts for lumps, rolling the breast tissue between your fingers.

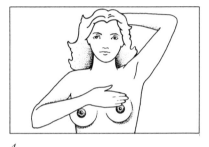

4.
Press against the chest wall to find any lumps that may be fixed to it.

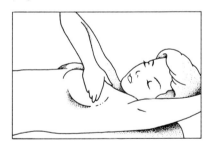

5.
Repeat the exam while lying down.

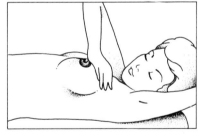

6.
Be sure to check in the armpit, as the tail of the breast tissue extends upward into this area.

All women should do a breast self-examination once a month. The best time to do it is following your menstrual period. Most women have some glandular nodules in their breasts; you will get used to your own glandular structure, so that you will know when a change occurs.

thorough inspection of the breast for dimpling or indentations, the breast tissue should be carefully rolled between two fingers feeling for hard areas (see accompanying illustration). Many women will feel some glandular tissue around the nipples. Tumors are usually hard and matted down in surrounding tissues, while fibromas are often rounded and freely mobile; but any mass should be evaluated by a physician.

Breast cancer, too, has a staging system. Except for very advanced, inoperable cases, treatment usually consists of one of the forms of radical mastectomy or, more recently, simple mastectomy or wide local excision, and radiation treatments.

The treatment of breast cancer remains one of the most hotly debated topics in medicine today. Although breast tumors have been described since very early times, only with the past century have surgeons aggressively tried to remove the disease. One commonly used operation in America is the Halsted radical mastectomy, which consists of complete removal of the breast, underlying chest wall muscles, and armpit lymph nodes. Another form of radical mastectomy, the Urban procedure, adds removal of the internal mammary chain of lymph nodes in the central chest wall. Following these procedures many women have some degree of limitation in their use of the arm that is affected, often accompanied by swelling (lymphedema) of the arm due to poor lymphatic drainage. Most women find the cosmetic defect of missing chest musculature extremely distressing, but many surgeons feel very strongly that radical mastectomy is by far the best treatment for breast cancer and that any less radical procedure is inadequate.

However, a few years ago, while most American centers were doing radical mastectomies, several surgeons in the United States and Europe essayed less disfiguring procedures. R. McWhirter in Great Britain, and W. George Crile, Jr., in the United States, among others, started to produce statistics showing that patients undergoing simple mastectomy and follow-up radiation therapy had very similar survival rates to those receiving radical mastectomy. F. Baclesse in France even advocated radiation alone. Some medical centers were in favor of simple lumpectomy (removal of the cancer mass), leaving the remainder of the breast intact. Obviously most women would prefer to have as limited an excision as possible, and the prospect of having only breast tissue removed, rather than chest-wall muscles as well, prompted many women to cheer the possibility of simple mastectomy.

But the controversy was far from over, and it still rages today. Arguments about patient selection, randomization and surgical variations in the published statistical studies have mired the results to the point that no clear-cut conclusions can be drawn about the various methods of treatment. All that can be said now is that some form of radical mastectomy remains a common treatment for breast cancer. More and more medical centers are moving toward simple mastectomy combined with radiation as their predominant treatment method. As yet, no clear-cut survival advantage has been demonstrated for either treatment.

In several areas the medical management of breast cancer has come a long way. Years back, most surgeons advocated biopsy under anesthesia so that a frozen section could be prepared for immediate tissue diagnosis, followed by immediate radical mastectomy if a malignancy was found. Women often awoke from the operation to find themselves without a breast before they even knew they had a malignancy. And even today some women prefer this rapid-fire surgical approach, which lifts all responsibility for decision making from their shoulders. But a more common practice now is to perform breast biopsy under local anesthesia. If the sample shows malignancy, the patient has a few days to adjust to the knowledge and to consider the options. Many women prefer such an adjustment period, which allows them time to explore their own feelings and those of their partners, and possibly to seek further opinions if their own doctor rigidly adheres to a type of treatment that the patient feels is not acceptable to her.

A second area in which medicine has come a long way is reconstructive surgery, or mammoplasty. Surgeons used to resist breast reconstruction on the grounds that the coverup material might make a recurrence of the cancer harder to detect. Besides, the mutilated chest-wall tissue made mammoplasty difficult and results were often poor. But today, greatly improved surgical materials and techniques, as well as evidence of the tremendous psychological benefits to many women, have persuaded more and more surgeons to do breast reconstructions. Nevertheless, since mammoplasty has not yet been perfected, many surgeons still resist the growing demand for breast reconstruction following mastectomy.

At some centers, surgeons do reconstructive work at the time of the original surgery; others prefer to perform reconstruction after a few weeks or months. A word of warning: If you do have mammoplasty following a breast-cancer operation, you should not expect miracles; an implant is not going to look or feel 100 percent normal. But the majority of women having breast reconstruction find their psychological adjustment much easier when the cosmetic defect of a missing breast is reduced. Other women adjust fairly well to their loss and do not feel the need for reconstruction, but any woman who is facing a mastectomy or who has had a mastectomy should certainly consider the possibility of breast reconstruction to ease the trauma of a changed body image.

Another word of warning: A few insurance companies have been reluctant to pay for mammoplasty, considering it "cosmetic" rather than "reconstructive" surgery. You'd be well advised to check with your insurance company *before* you run up a large hospital bill.

You may have noticed that the subjects of mammography, xeroradiography (a photoelectric process) and thermography were conspicuously absent from the above discussion of diagnosis of breast cancer. Despite much fanfare and a few avid advocates of these specialized procedures, they have not come into widespread use for several reasons. First, they are not very sensitive in detection —that is, each technique may miss a fair proportion of tumors. Second, they are not very specific—i.e., each technique may reveal lesions that are not tumors. Finally, mammography and xeroradiography, which are specialized x-ray techniques, may themselves add to cancer risk through increased x-ray exposure. Thermography, which simply detects "hot" areas of breast tissue, can often detect tumors, since cancerous tissue usually has a higher metabolic rate and hence be "hotter" than surrounding tissue. Thus thermography, when it becomes more refined and specific, may prove to be a superbly useful diagnostic aid. Other promising techniques include ultrasound evaluation of breast tissue (bouncing sound waves off masses in a manner somewhat similar to radar) and Pap-smear-type studies of breast secretion.

Many physicians recommend mammograms for women with

breast lumps or women at risk of developing breast cancer. Some physicians recommend mammography for any woman over age fifty. The American College of Obstetricians and Gynecologists limits the risk factors that would call for mammograms to the following: Mass or nipple discharge; previous breast surgery; disease in the other breast; strong family history of breast cancer; first pregnancy after the age of thirty; and masses scheduled for surgery. While mammograms do have a place in these special circumstances, we are not yet ready to use them routinely, as questions of reliability, cost-effectiveness and safety have not all been answered. But mammography is a rapidly developing field and in the future may be as reliable and safe as the Pap test.

More and more attention is being focused not on surgery but on either chemotherapy or radiation therapy. There is a great deal of misunderstanding about what adjunctive therapy is supposed to offer. In a few rare circumstances, such as some early cervical carcinomas, adjunctive therapy can be curative, but as a rule it is either palliative (intended to slow down the course of tumor growth) or prophylactic (intended to prevent regrowth of a tumor that has been largely removed). Both chemotherapy and radiation therapy have been found useful in some types of tumors, sometimes apparently producing a cure. More often they delay growth of a tumor that is too large to be entirely removed by surgery.

Chemotherapy

Chemotherapy means treatment of disease by chemical agents. Useful chemotherapeutic agents harm disease organisms or diseased tissues more than they harm healthy tissues. An antibiotic such as penicillin destroys the cell membranes of many types of bacteria while doing very little harm to normal human cells. But differences between human cells and bacterial cells are substantial, whereas those between cancer cells and normal human cells are very slight. As a result, cancer chemotherapeutic drugs must either depend on these very small differences between body cells or do the same damage to normal cells as to cancer cells.

Most chemotherapy used in cancer treatment interferes with the growth and multiplication of cells. Since cancer cells often multiply

at a rate much faster than normal body cells, any agent that interferes with this process may slow down or stop tumor growth. A few
chemotherapy agents cut off vitamins necessary to cell growth,
hence preventing normal growth and multiplication of cancer cells.

What does this mean in practical terms? It means that chemotherapy can prevent growth and multiplication of all normal cells as well
as of tumor cells. Fortunately, in adults many body systems do not
depend on multiplication of cells. But the side effects of chemotherapy are mostly on those tissues that normally contain rapidly dividing cells. Thus, the very distressing side effects of hair loss, various
stomach and intestinal disturbances, and skin changes can occur.
The most serious effects from a medical point of view are on the
blood-building system; production of blood requires a continuous
manufacture of new cells in the bone marrow. White cells (which
fight infection) and platelets (which help to clot blood) are the most
drastically affected; the red cells that carry oxygen to tissues may
also be affected, causing anemia. The kidneys and bladder are particularly sensitive to some types of chemotherapy, because the drugs
become concentrated in these organs for excretion. Other types of
chemotherapy may cause problems such as weakness of the heart
muscle, lung fibrosis or nerve weakness.

Hormonal chemotherapy has proved extremely useful for some
cancers. Some tumors—most commonly breast, endometrial and
ovarian carcinomas—have what are called "receptors" for various
hormones. Sometimes exposure to estrogen from the body seems to
stimulate tumor growth. Either "blocking" androgens (male hormones) or "estrogen antagonists" may be used to eliminate this
estrogen stimulation, stopping tumor progress almost entirely. Side
effects are less serious than with traditional cancer chemotherapy,
since most body tissues do not depend to a great extent on estrogen
receptors for normal function.

Radiation Therapy

Radiotherapy is the use of either x-rays or radioactive materials to
treat disease. X-rays or radioactive substances interfere with cell
growth by interfering with the DNA-RNA structure (the genetic
material of a cell that must be duplicated to form new cells or to

manufacture proteins for cellular function). One major advantage of radiation therapy is that x-ray beams may be focused on specific tissues rather than being diffused all over the body cells, as happens in chemotherapy. Furthermore, x-rays aimed at an area surrounding a tumor can eradicate clusters of tumor cells too small to be seen and removed surgically.

The disadvantage of radiotherapy is that it affects all the cells in its pathway. As in chemotherapy, rapidly reproducing cells are those most seriously affected. Also, radiation causes some scarring and fibrosis of the tissues it affects.

The most common instances of radiation therapy for gynecologic malignancies are external radiation, such as a cobalt or neutron beam, used for breast, cervical or uterine cancers, and implants of radioactive materials into the vagina for cervical cancers. Skin cancers, including vulvar cancers, are often treated with external radiation. Radiation can also be useful if a tumor is pressing on a vital structure. Often, treatment can shrink the mass enough to allow normal function of the involved structure.

Side effects of radiation treatments result from the scarring and fibrosis of nearby tissues and organs, and damage to actively rebuilding tissues. In radiation to the pelvic area, side effects may be diarrhea from damage to the bowel, radiation cystitis causing blood in the urine, and even breakdown of the tissues between bladder, vagina and rectum, causing fistulas, or openings. Fortunately the majority of women receiving pelvic radiation do not have the worst side effects; many women have diarrhea during treatment, which can be controlled with medicines and usually improves when treatments are finished. Since the pelvic bones are active in the production of blood cells, there usually is some decrease in the body's ability to produce red and white blood cells, but in a milder form than with chemotherapy, since not all blood-producing bones are affected.

Although tissue fibrosis and poor circulation in the affected arm can result from radiation treatments of a diseased breast, the side effects from radiation are usually minor compared to the tissue scarring and circulatory problems that can result from radical breast surgery. Results are not yet clear on the long-range effects of radiation therapy in combination with simpler surgical procedures for breast cancer, and although the subject is still highly controversial, the trend seems to be toward the use of less aggressive surgery and more aggressive radiation therapy in the treatment of breast cancer.

Cancer certainly deserves its position as the disease Americans dread the most. But not all cancers are disastrous; thanks to the increased use of Pap smears, breast exam and endometrial sampling procedures, many gynecologic malignancies are discovered in the early stages and cured. For people who must live with the knowledge of having cancer, many treatment alternatives are available; unfortunately many cancers still cannot be cured.

Having a malignancy does not make a person different. We are all made of material with a limited time to survive. The person with a malignancy is only more acutely aware of how transient all of life is; she must make a little more effort to appreciate each day.

EPILOGUE

We said at the beginning of this book that no woman in our society today lives in the same world as her mother did; and this was never more true than at the present moment, in the latter years of the twentieth century.

What we have tried to give you in this book is not merely a course in general and gynecologic physiology but a point of view: that understanding your body and taking effective care of it are major conditions for getting the most out of life, and that today as never before, women have both the opportunity and the responsibility to be "well" in the fullest sense.

We believe that knowing your body leads to confidence and skill in its care, increases your well-being and vitality, and adds greater depth, force and beauty to your life.

We also believe that more knowledge means less fear and uncertainty about ourselves. Knowledge helps us dispel the destructive myths that, alas, still haunt society—the myths about the essential "sickliness" of the feminine reproductive functions: menstruation, pregnancy, childbirth and the menopause.

We have made a special effort to bring you useful information that will help you to understand and work with your doctor—information that will enable you to distinguish those things a physician can do for you from those things you can do for yourself.

We hope this book has both increased your understanding of the female body and eliminated some health worries and problems for you. A point we wish to emphasize to the younger woman is that while health care now brings its prompt rewards in feeling fine and functioning well, the care you give your youthful body is most important as an investment for the future—the way you will look, feel and function in your fifties, sixties and beyond.

For the older woman, the importance of maintaining active health increases as the years pass. Today we are seeing a kind of renaissance in the activities, achievements and creative powers of older people, to whom aging is a totally different experience than it was even a generation ago. We have tried in this book to support this trend by showing the phases of a woman's physical life and what her normal expectations are for continuing health and vitality.

Along the way, we hope we have shared with you a sense of wonder at the structure and workings of the female human body.

GLOSSARY

cholesterol	A pearly fatty substance found in many body tissues and in foods of animal origin; actually a form of alcohol.
climacteric	The time of life that occurs around the end of the reproductive period.
clitoris	The small, erectile organ at the entrance of the vagina.
condyloma acuminata	Genital wart.
corpus luteum	The follicle in the ovary that has released its egg. If conception has taken place, it enlarges and secretes progesterone for several months; if not, it shrinks and disappears about the time of menstruation.
cystitis	Inflammation of the urinary bladder.

D

diagnosis	The art of distinguishing one disease or condition from another and determining its nature.
dilation and curettage (D&C)	The use of instruments to enlarge the cervical opening and to scrape the inner surface of the uterus.
dysmenorrhea	Painful menstruation.
dysplasia	Abnormal cells that are found in tissue which may possibly progress to cancer.

E

ectopic (pregnancy)	"Out of place"; in pregnancy, usually a fetus growing inside a Fallopian tube.
elective (surgery)	Any necessary or desirable surgery that is not an emergency.
endometriosis	Tissue like that of the uterine lining, growing elsewhere in the abdominal cavity.
endometrium	The tissue that lines the uterus.
enzyme	A substance that causes chemical changes in other substances, such as changing starch into sugar.

F

Fallopian tubes	Slender tubes through which the egg is transported from the ovary to the uterus.

G

gestation	Period of fetal growth and development between conception and birth.

H

human chorionic gonadotropin (HCG)	A hormone produced by the placenta during pregnancy that has a stimulating effect on organs of reproduction. May be measured in blood or urine and forms the basis of most pregnancy tests.
herpesvirus	A virus causing blisters on the lips, skin or genital tissues.
hymen	A fold of tissue that may partly or completely close the vaginal opening. Also called the "maidenhead."
hyperplasia	Abnormal increase of cells in an organ such as the uterus.

I

intrauterine device (IUD)	Small plastic object placed in the uterus for contraceptive purposes. May be shaped like a loop, L, T, or 7; may emit progestin or copper ions.

L

labia	"Lips"; in the vulva, the labia major a are the outer folds, labia minor a the inner folds at the vaginal opening.
lesion	A break in tissue or in a part of the body.

M

mastectomy	Excision or removal of the breast.
masturbation	Self-stimulation of the genitalia to produce orgasm.
menarche	The beginning of menstruation.
menorrhagia	Excessive menstrual bleeding.
menstruation	Normal, cyclic bleeding from the uterus.
metrorrhagia	Uterine bleeding at irregular intervals.
Mittelschmerz	Abdominal pain or discomfort due to ovulation.
multiparous	Having had two or more pregnancies.

O

oligomenorrhea	Scanty or infrequent menstruation.
osteoporosis	Thinning and softening of the bones.
ovulation	Release of an egg from the ovary.

P

placenta

A membranous, temporary endocrine organ inside the uterus, connecting the mother and fetus by means of the umbilical cord. Known commonly as "afterbirth."

polyp

Any growth protruding from a mucous membrane.

prognosis

Physician's estimate of the course of a disease or condition, based on all available information.

prostaglandin

A simple body chemical substance with many different effects, particularly on smooth muscle contraction and blood-vessel dilation.

S

sign

An indication of a condition or disease, or objective evidence of a body change that can be demonstrated to others.

Skene's glands

Ducts that drain other glands in the urethra, or urinary tube.

sperm (spermatozoa)

Male reproductive cells.

STD

See *venereal disease.*

steroids

Fat-soluble organic compounds, such as bile, sex hormones, etc.

suction curettage

Clearing surface tissues and contents of the uterus with a vacuum instrument instead of a curette. Also called aspiration curettage.

symptom

Evidence of a condition or a disease, or a change from normal function, as experienced by the patient.

U

urinary-tract infection (UTI)

Any infection that involves the bladder, urethra or kidneys.

V

vaginitis

Inflammation of the vagina, usually with pain and discharge.

venereal disease (VD)

Several kinds of contagious diseases involving the reproductive tract, usually transmitted by sexual contact but capable of passing from mother to unborn or newborn child. Today venereal diseases are usually included in the larger class of sexually transmitted diseases (STDs).

vulva   The external female genital structures, comprising the labia minora, labia majora, mons pubis, clitoris, perineum and vaginal vestibule.

PERSONAL HISTORY

Medical Problems

Date	Nature of Illness	Physician	Comments (status of illness)
SAMPLE 9/76	High Blood Pressure	Smith	

Hospitalization

Date	Hospital	Reason	Description (type of surgery)
SAMPLE 7/62	Western Community Hospital	Appendicitis	Appendectomy

Gynecologic History (including childbirth)

Age at First Period	Normal Cycle Length (days)	Frequency (days)	Menopause (if applicable)	Comments
SAMPLE 12	5	29	47	

Date of Deliveries	Type	Weight of Child	Health of Child	Comments
SAMPLE 1970	vaginal	8 lbs	good	

Medications You Take

Name	Date	Dose	Frequency
SAMPLE aspirin	started 1975	up to 4 a day	when arthritis flares

Allergies

Date	Nature of Allergy	Reaction
SAMPLE 1971	penicillin	rash

DISEASES OF YOUR BLOOD RELATIONS

	Serious Illness	Age at Death	Cause of Death
Mother			
Father			
Grandparents (Maternal)			
Grandparents (Paternal)			
Brothers/Sisters			
Other (Aunts, Uncles, Cousins)			

INDEX

granuloma inguinale, *see* Sexually Transmitted Diseases
Guttmacher, Alan 109
Gwinup, Grant 6
gynecologic infections
  abdominal pain 175–190
  Bartholin's glands 154
  oral sex 140
  pelvic infections 182–183
  sexually transmitted diseases 140–142, 148–153
  Skene's glands 154
  toxic shock syndrome 72, 181–182
  vaginitis 140–148, 156
  venereal warts 154–155
  See also Sexually Transmitted Diseases; Vaginitis 140–156
gynecologists 33

Halsted radical mastectomy 232
headaches 44–45, 57
  migraine 45, 114–115
  premenstrual tension 175–176
health habits
  bad habits 31–32
  body care 29–31
  diet 20–27
  exercise 27–29
  sleep 29
Heaney, Robert P. 208
hearing
  aging 201–202
heart
  aging 200–201
  circulatory system 4, 12–14
heart disease 9, 12–14, 114
  alcohol 31–32
  and exercise 27
  palpitations 55
  smoking 31
  syphilis 151
heartburn, *see* Indigestion
hematoma 121
hemophilus vaginalis, *see* Vaginitis
hemorrhage, *see* Bleeding; Pregnancy—Ectopic
hemorrhoids 49, 53, 79, 229
hepatitis 43, 174
hernias 184
herpes, *see* Sexually Transmitted Diseases
high blood pressure, *see* Hypertension
high-density lipoprotein (HDL), *see* Foods and Nutrition—cholesterol
home birth 81, 101
home pregnancy test kits 82, 112
hormones 159, 164
  androgen 5, 66, 75–76
  chemotherapy 236

depression 55
  during menstruation 70, 73
endometriosis 176
estrogen 5, 50, 65–66, 73, 76–78, 114–115, 177, 197, 213, 225–226, (illus.) 67
  and heart disease 13
follicle-stimulating hormone 66–67, 135, (illus.) 67
human chorionic gonadatropin 82, 136
infertility 133, 135–138
luteinizing hormone 66–67, 135, 137, (illus.) 67
male 8, 66, 75–76
oral contraceptives 114–115, 128–129
progesterone 111–112, 114–115
progestin 66, 69
prostaglandins 73, 76, 126, 129, 175
testosterone 8
hospitals
  birthing rooms 100
  intensive care nurseries 98
  interns and residents 170
  maternity wards 100
  routine tests 169
hot flashes, *see* Menopause
HSV, *see* Sexually Transmitted Diseases
Human Life and Natural Family Planning Foundation 105–106
hydrotubation 137
hymen 71
  infertility 133
hyperplasia 77–78
hypertension 114, 225
  headaches 44–45, 57
  heart disease 12–13
  salt 25
hyperthyroidism 43–44
hypothyroidism 42–44
hysterectomy 62, 77, 117, 157–163, 166, 171–172, 176, 178, 182, 188–189, 224, 228
hysterotomy, *see* Abortion

impotence, *see* Men
incontinence, *see* Urinary Tract
indigestion 47–48, 57
  from milk 91
  gas pains 174, 178
  ulcers 174
infants
  candidiasis 145–146
  chlamydial infections 147
  venereal disease 149
infections—gynecologic, *see* Gynecologic Infections
infertility 132–139
  adoption 139
  artificial insemination 138–139

ABOUT THE AUTHORS

LINDA HUGHEY HOLT, M.D., born in Chicago and reared in Wilmette, Illinois, was one of the first women to attend Yale University, where she became interested in the problems of women's health care. Dr. Holt received her undergraduate degree in English Literature from Yale and then entered the University of Chicago Pritzker School of Medicine, where she completed medical school and a residency program in obstetrics-gynecology. .

Dr. Holt currently works for a health-maintenance organization in the Chicago area and is on the clinical teaching staff of Noṛthwestern University School of Medicine. She has also served with the Indian Health Service.

Dr. Holt is married to a faculty member at the University of Chicago.

MELVA WEBER writes frequently on subjects of medicine and health care, with special emphasis on women's interests. She is the medical writer for *Vogue* magazine and author of the publication's monthly "*Vogue* Health" page. In addition, Ms. Weber is a science writer at the National Cancer Institute in Bethesda, Maryland. She worked previously as a writer in New York for *Medical World News*, a magazine for physicians.

Ms. Weber is a native of Mount Auburn, Iowa, and received undergraduate degrees in journalism and English literature from the University of Iowa in Iowa City. She lives in Arlington, Virginia.

BOBBYE COCHRAN is a free-lance illustrator whose work ranges from medical publications to children's books, animation, design and advertising. Born in New Albany, Indiana, Ms. Cochran received her bachelor of fine arts degree from Washington University in St. Louis. She has won awards for her work in both the United States and Europe.

DEMCO